Manual of Nutrition

Tenth Edition

London: TSO

TSO

Published by TSO (The Stationery Office) and available from:

Online
www.tso.co.uk/bookshop

Mail, Telephone, Fax & E-mail
TSO
PO Box 29, Norwich NR3 1GN
Telephone orders/General enquiries: 0870 600 5522
Fax orders: 0870 600 5533
E-mail: book.orders@tso.co.uk
Textphone: 0870 240 3701

TSO Shops
123 Kingsway, London WC2B 6PQ
020 7242 6393 Fax 020 7242 6394
68-69 Bull Street, Birmingham B4 6AD
0121 236 9696 Fax 0121 236 9699
9-21 Princess Street, Manchester M60 8AS
0161 834 7201 Fax 0161 833 0634
16 Arthur Street, Belfast BT1 4GD
028 9023 8451 Fax 028 9023 5401
18-19 High Street, Cardiff CF10 1PT
029 2039 5548 Fax 029 2038 4347
71 Lothian Road, Edinburgh EH3 9AZ
0870 606 5566 Fax 0870 606 5588

TSO Accredited Agents
(see Yellow Pages)

and through good booksellers

Contents

List of tables

Foreword

The tenth edition of the *Manual of Nutrition* is published at a time when there is continuing interest in the relationships between food and health and increasing efforts are being made towards improvements in the health of the nation. There is particular concern about fat, sugar, salt and dietary fibre, but the science of nutrition is much broader than that. This manual therefore describes all the important nutrients, their roles in the body, the foods that provide them, and the way in which these foods are digested so that the nutrients can be utilised by the body.

As in the previous edition, this manual goes on to describe the effects of cooking and processing on each nutrient, and the nutritional principles involved in choosing a healthy balanced diet and in evaluating eating habits. There are also sections on the special nutritional needs of different sections of the population and how they can be met, and on the new Dietary Reference Values. Finally there are appendices which give up-to-date values for the typical nutrient content of a wide range of common foods, describe EC and UK legislation affecting the nutrient content of foods and their labelling, and give suggestions for further reading.

Grateful thanks go to Jennifer Woolfe for preparation of this edition, to Alison Mills, Gillian Smithers, Cecilia McGrath, Sejal Patel and Katherine Newall for technical assistance with the tables, and to Janet Lewis, David Buss and Martin Wiseman for scientific advice.

Food Standards Agency

PART 1

Nutrients and their utilisation

1 Introduction to nutrition, and some definitions

In other countries many of the foods eaten are very different from our own, yet the majority of their people grow well and stay healthy provided that they get enough to eat. The reasons for this, and the ways in which the adequacy of any diet can be assessed, form part of the science of nutrition with which this manual is concerned. A knowledge of its principles is thus important to all of us, but especially to those who plan and provide meals.

Before proceeding further, it is necessary to define some terms:

The science of *nutrition* is the study of all processes of growth, maintenance and repair of the living body which depend upon the digestion of food, and the study of that food.

Food is any solid or liquid which when swallowed can supply any of the following:

(a) material from which the body can produce movement, heat or other forms of energy
(b) material for growth, repair or reproduction
(c) substances necessary to regulate the production of energy or the processes of growth and repair.

Foods are considered in more detail in Part 2.

The components of foods which have these functions are called *nutrients*. They are introduced below, and considered in more detail in Chapters 2, 3, 4, 7 and 8. The *diet* consists of those foods or mixtures of foods in the amounts which are actually eaten (usually each day). A good diet will provide adequate amounts of all the nutrients, without harmful excesses, from a wide range of foods.

The nutrients in food

The following types of nutrients may be present in foods:

Carbohydrates, which provide the body with energy, and may also be converted into body fat.

Fats, which provide energy in a more concentrated form than carbohydrates, and may also be converted into body fat.

Proteins, which provide materials (amino acids) for growth and repair. They can also be converted into carbohydrate and used to provide energy.

1

Minerals, which are used in growth and repair, and help to regulate body processes.

Vitamins, which help to regulate body processes.[1]

Although water, like oxygen from the air, is also essential for life, it is not usually considered as a food or a nutrient. The group of carbohydrate compounds, known collectively as 'fibre', are not strictly nutrients but have positive effects on our health. On the other hand, alcohol would be considered a food because it provides energy, even though it has drug-like properties. Iron from a cooking utensil is also a nutrient since it may be used to renew substances in the blood.

Hardly any foods contain only one nutrient. Most are very complex mixtures, which consist mainly of a variety of carbohydrates, fats and proteins, together with water. Minerals and vitamins are present in very much smaller amounts. One hundred grams (g) of potatoes, for example, contain about 18 g carbohydrates, 2 g proteins, 80 g water and some fibre, but less than 50 mg of minerals and vitamins (and if fried they will also contain fat).

Energy

Energy is needed for the body to function and be active. The body derives energy from carbohydrates, fat, protein and alcohol in the diet. Experiments show that almost exactly the same amount of energy is produced from, say, wheat when it is eaten by humans as when it is used for fuel in a railway engine (as it has been in times of glut). The essential difference between the two chemical processes is that in the body the energy is released gradually by a series of steps, each carefully controlled by an enzyme.[2] This energy is used to perform muscular work and to maintain body temperature and such processes as breathing, but a considerable amount is also lost as heat. The energy provided by carbohydrate, fat, protein and other constituents can be measured and used to calculate the energy value of any food (see p. 30).

Other constituents of food

WATER

Water comprises about two-thirds of the body's weight, and is the medium or solvent in which almost every body process takes place both inside and outside the cells. The need of the body for water is second only to its need for

---

[1] *Vitamins* differ from hormones (which also help to regulate body processes) in that, with the exception of vitamin D, they cannot be made in the body and must therefore be supplied in the diet; hormones are always made within the body itself.

[2] *Enzymes* are special proteins, each of which accelerates the rate of a specific chemical reaction without itself being affected. They enable complex changes to occur in the body that would otherwise require more extreme conditions; without them life could not exist. Many require the presence of vitamins or minerals as 'co-factors' in order to act.

air: adults can survive for many weeks without food but for only a few days without water. Water comes from solid foods as well as from drinks (p. 132), and it is lost by evaporation in the breath and sweat as well as in the urine. The balance of water retained in the body is normally very carefully regulated by the kidneys, but excessive losses can result from vomiting or diarrhoea in illness or from heavy sweating due to strenuous activity or a hot climate. Then, if water intake is not increased, dehydration may result. In temperate climates at least 1 litre (2 pints) of water or other fluid should be drunk each day; more will be needed if heavy work is done.

FIBRE

Some foods, particularly wholegrain cereals, pulses and some fruit and vegetables, contain substantial amounts of fibre (non-starch polysaccharides – see p. 133). Insoluble fibre fractions are not absorbed into the body; instead they add bulk to the faeces. This property is beneficial to health, in helping to prevent constipation. Soluble fibre constituents, which may be absorbed, are found especially in fruit, vegetables and pulses and can help to reduce the amount of cholesterol in the blood. However, fibre can also decrease the absorption of certain nutrients – especially some of the minerals. Fibre is further discussed on p. 7.

FLAVOURS AND COLOURS

In addition to the main nutritive and structural components, foods also contain innumerable minor constituents which give them their characteristic flavours, colours and textures. Control over the changes which occur in these constituents after ripening, and during storage, preparation and cooking, is an important consideration for both cooks and food technologists.

Malnutrition

The maintenance of health in an individual depends upon the consumption and absorption of appropriate amounts of energy and all the nutrients. Too little or too much of some, usually over a period of months or longer, may lead to ill health or malnutrition. Although the body has considerable power to adapt to reduced dietary intakes, for example by reduced physical activity, too low an intake of food will eventually result in *undernutrition* and, in extreme cases, *starvation*. An example is the wasting (marasmus) in young children and stunting of physical and perhaps even mental development, which may result from inadequate breast feeding or from a poor weaning diet in developing countries. Other examples include the 'classical' nutrition deficiency diseases such as scurvy and some anaemias which result from diets containing too little of one or more minerals or vitamins, or from a physiological inability to absorb these nutrients. Excessive fatness (obesity), resulting from too great a food intake for the body's needs, is also a form of malnutrition, as is the excessive consumption of any nutrient, whether fat, sugar, mineral or vitamin, if it leads to ill health.

Units of measurement

Standard units are used to calculate the energy and nutrients in various amounts of food, and to measure heights and weights. The metric system (including the form known as SI[3]) has mainly been used in this edition of the manual. The relationships between these and traditional units are given in some detail in Appendix 1.

---

[3] This system mainly affects the definition of energy, which has been measured in *kilocalories* (1 kcal being the amount of heat required to raise the temperature of 1 kg of water by 1°C). The SI unit, the *joule*, is hard to define in familiar terms, but 1 *kilojoule* (kJ) may be visualised as the amount of heat required to raise the temperature of 239 g of water by 1°C. 1 *megajoule* (1 MJ) = 1000 kJ.

2 Carbohydrates

There are three major groups of carbohydrates in food: *sugars, starches* and *non-starch polysaccharides* (NSP). All are compounds of carbon, hydrogen and oxygen only, and their chemical structures are all based on a common unit (usually glucose). The units can be linked together in varying ways and in different numbers, and classification of the carbohydrates depends primarily on the number of units which varies from one to many thousands. Sugars and starches are a major source of food energy for humans throughout the world. Non-starch polysaccharides are known collectively as *fibre* ('dietary fibre').

Sugars

MONOSACCHARIDES (OR SIMPLE SUGARS)
Glucose (dextrose) occurs naturally in fruit and plant juices and in the blood of living animals. Most carbohydrates in food are ultimately converted to glucose during digestion. Glucose can also be manufactured from starch by the action of acid or specific enzymes. *Glucose syrups* (liquid glucose) result from the hydrolysis of starch (usually maize or wheat starch), and contain variable concentrations of glucose, maltose and various more complex carbohydrates depending on the end use for which they are intended. Except where the syrup is almost pure glucose, these syrups are less sweet than glucose. They are used in many manufactured foods including sugar confectionery, soft drinks and jams. Dried glucose is also made for domestic and industrial use.

Fructose occurs naturally in some fruit and vegetables and especially in honey. It is the sweetest sugar known. It is also a component of sucrose, from which it may be derived. The conversion of some of the glucose in glucose syrup to fructose results in the production of 'high fructose' syrups.

Galactose occurs mainly as part of lactose, but can be found in the free state in some foods.

DISACCHARIDES
Disaccharides consist of two monosaccharides linked together (minus the elements of water).

Sucrose occurs naturally in sugar cane and sugar beet, and in lesser amounts in fruits and some root vegetables such as carrots. It is a chemical combination of glucose and fructose. 'Sugar', whether white or brown, is essentially pure sucrose.

Maltose is formed during the breakdown of starch by digestion and, for example, when grain is germinated for the production of malt liquors such as beer. It is a combination of two glucose units.

Lactose occurs only in milk, including human milk. It is less sweet than sucrose or glucose, and is a combination of glucose and galactose. It is added in an isolated form to some food products including meat products and some infant foods.

Properties of sugars

All sugars, whether monosaccharides or disaccharides, dissolve in water but vary in sweetness. Their taste may be modified by cooking (e.g. by caramelization). They usually form white (colourless) crystals when the water in which they are dissolved becomes supersaturated, but impure preparations may be brown. In addition to sweetness they provide a readily available source of energy; monosaccharides provide 16 kJ (3.75 kcal) per gram and disaccharides 17 kJ (4 kcal) per gram. Sugars can be used for several purposes in food preparation. For example, in jam-making and bottling they act as preservatives, and in biscuits, cakes, soft drinks and certain other foods, they also help to provide the characteristic texture and consistency.

Non-sugar sweeteners

Some other substances also taste sweet. *Sorbitol, mannitol* and *xylitol* are polyols (also known as sugar alcohols) which are made from sugars. They are sometimes used in diabetic foods because they are absorbed only slowly. Their energy value is similar to that of glucose, but for labelling purposes they are deemed to provide 10 kJ (2.4 kcal) per gram. In contrast, the intense sweeteners saccharin, aspartame and acesulfame K are classed as food additives as they have no chemical or nutritional relationship to sugars. They are about 200–500 times as sweet as sucrose and consequently used at a very low level so that even aspartame, which is the only one metabolised by the body, provides essentially no energy. They may be used as sweetening agents when it is desirable to restrict the amount of sugar in the diet. Certain sweetening agents available in a granulated form (for example to sprinkle on breakfast cereals) are mixtures of an intense sweetener and a carbohydrate diluent and as such are sources of energy, although substantially less than the equivalent amount of sugar.

Starch

There are a number of starches, which are *polysaccharides* composed of variably large numbers of glucose units linked together to form both straight and branched chains (*amylose* and *amylopectin*, respectively). They exist in granules of a size and shape which are characteristic for each plant. In this form they are insoluble in water, and foods such as flour and potatoes, which contain large amounts of them, are indigestible if eaten raw. When heated or cooked in the presence of water, the starch granules swell and eventually gelatinise. They can then be more easily digested. One gram of starch provides approximately 17.6 kJ (4.2 kcal) of energy, but for food labelling purposes a value of 17 kJ (4 kcal) is used. Some forms of processing, for example dry heat used in the manufacture of certain breakfast cereals, can make part of the starch indigestible. Some scientists regard this fraction, known as *resistant starch*, as fibre along with non-starch polysaccharides (see below).

Glycogen is similar to starch in composition, but is made from glucose only by animals and not by plants. Small amounts are stored in the liver and muscles as an energy reserve. It is not a significant item in the diet because it breaks down again to glucose after an animal's death.

Non-starch polysaccharides (NSP)

In addition to starch there are other polysaccharides found in the cell walls of vegetables, fruits, pulses and cereal grains where they provide part of the plant structure. This range of diverse compounds, when forming part of the human diet, is classified as *fibre* (Table 2). The non-starch polysaccharides in wheat, maize and rice are mainly insoluble cellulose and related materials, but those in fruits, vegetables and the cereals oats, barley and rye also contain soluble forms including pectins and gums.

Cellulose consists of many thousands of glucose units. It cannot be digested by humans, but can be used as food by cows and other ruminants whose digestive tract contains microorganisms capable of breaking it down into glucose. Cellulose and other indigestible polysaccharides add bulk to the faeces because of their water-binding capacity, and greatly assist the passage of digestible materials and waste products through the intestines, thus helping to prevent constipation.

Pectin is present in apples and many other fruits and in roots such as turnips and sweetpotatoes. Its property of forming a stiff jelly is important in jam-making. Pectin is not fibrous, and because it is completely digested it has little effect on the faeces. However, pectin and other soluble fibre components can help to reduce the amount of cholesterol in the blood.

As the effects of both soluble and insoluble NSP are beneficial, it is best to include a variety of NSP-rich foods in the diet. Intakes of NSP in the UK average about 12 g per day, being provided mainly by vegetables and cereals. It has been recommended, however, that average intakes of NSP should rise to 18 g per day (see p. 72).

Fibre components can bind minerals such as calcium, iron, copper and zinc making them unavailable to the body. However, the only people likely to be adversely affected by high-fibre diets are those who have a low or marginal mineral intake.

Sources of carbohydrates in the diet

Plants form sugars in their leaves by the action of sunlight, but store them in their stems, roots, tubers or seeds as starch (the small amount of starch stored in unripe fruits, however, turns back into glucose or sucrose on ripening). Starch forms the major energy reserve of most plants, and thus in turn provides a major part of food energy for humans. The principal sources of sugar in the diet are milk (lactose), fruit and honey (fructose), sucrose, glucose syrups and fruit juices used both alone and in jams, canned fruit, cakes, biscuits, ice cream and other foods prepared in the home or by food manufacturers.

The sugar and starch content of selected foods is shown in Table 1. Twenty eight per cent of the present intake of carbohydrate in the UK consists of sucrose and glucose syrups (non-milk extrinsic sugars – see p. 10), 7 per cent is lactose, and the remainder, intrinsic sugars and starch. A century ago, flour and potato consumption was much higher and sucrose consumption much lower. Then, as in the developing countries now, starch was a much more important component of the diet. In 1997, however, total sugars provided almost the same percentage of dietary energy (21 per cent) as did starch (26 per cent). The total fibre content of the average UK diet has not changed much over the past century, but a greater proportion now comes from vegetables and less from cereals as a result of changing eating habits. There has, however, been an increase in recent years in the consumption of wholemeal bread and bran-containing breakfast cereals.

Health aspects of carbohydrates

Although all sugars and starches absorbed by the body provide similar amounts of energy, they have different physiological effects. Eating a lot of certain types of sugary foods at frequent intervals, especially between meals, is associated with increased tooth decay (dental caries). The Government's advisory Committee on Medical Aspects of Food and Nutrition Policy (COMA) consider that the type of sugar and its location within a food can

Table 1. Average carbohydrate content of selected foods (edible portion).

	Available carbohydrate, as monosaccharides		
	Sugars (g/100 g)	Starch (g/100 g)	Total (g/100 g)
Whole milk[a]	4.8	0.0	4.8
Skimmed milk	5.0	0.0	5.0
Ice cream (non-dairy)	23.1	Tr	23.1
Meat	0.0	0.0	0.0
Sugar[b]	105.0	0.0	105.0
Honey	76.4	0.0	76.4
Jam	69.0	0.0	69.0
Baked beans	5.9	9.4	15.3
Potatoes, old, boiled	0.7	16.3	17.0
Yam, boiled	0.7	32.3	33.0
Bananas	20.9	2.3	23.2
Oranges	8.5	0.0	8.5
Peaches canned in syrup	14.0	0.0	14.0
Peaches canned in juice	9.7	0.0	9.7
Sultanas	69.4	0.0	69.4
Biscuits, chocolate, fully coated	43.4	24.0	67.4
Bread, white	2.6	46.7	49.3
Bread, wholemeal	1.8	39.8	41.6
Flour, white	1.5	76.2	77.7
Cornflakes	8.2	77.7	85.9
Muesli, average (with added sugar)	26.2	46.0	72.2
Porridge oats	1.1	64.9	66.0
Fruit juice, unsweetened	8.8	0.0	8.8
Soft drink, carbonated	10.5	0.0	10.5
Soup, canned, tomato	2.6	3.3	5.9
Tomato ketchup	22.9	1.1	24.0
Milk chocolate	56.5	2.9	59.4
Lager	1.5	0.0	1.5
Wine, white, medium	3.4	0.0	3.4

[a] Lactose
[b] Equivalent to 100 g of sucrose
   1 g of disaccharide is equivalent to 1.05 g of monosaccharide.
   1 g of starch is equivalent to 1.10 g of monosaccharide.
The main sources of sugars in the diet are sugar, soft drinks, cakes and biscuits, fruit and fruit juice, milk (as lactose), sweets and chocolate. The main sources of starches in the diet are bread, potatoes, cakes, biscuits and other cereal products.

affect its ability to cause dental caries, and that it is useful to classify sugars in the following way:

Intrinsic sugars are those contained within the cell walls of food, e.g. sugars in whole fruits and vegetables.

Extrinsic sugars are those not contained within the cell structure of a food and include:

Milk sugars which occur naturally in milk and milk products (almost all lactose).

'*Non-milk extrinsic (NME) sugars*, e.g. sugars in fruit juices, table sugar, sugars added to food.'

Intrinsic and milk sugars are not considered by COMA to have adverse effects on teeth. NME sugars, on the other hand, can play a significant part in tooth decay, although this effect can be lessened by regular brushing of teeth and the use of fluoride toothpaste.

When it is desirable to reduce the fat content of the diet, a good way of replacing the lost energy is by increasing the intake of fibre-rich starchy foods. There are now targets for the amounts of NME, intrinsic and milk sugars, starch and NSP to be eaten on average by the population (see Chapter 9). NME sugars should contribute no more than 10 per cent of dietary energy on average for the population. In 1997, 13 per cent of dietary energy was consumed as NME sugars by the average person. In the same year, 34 per cent of dietary energy came from starch and other sugars, compared to the 37 per cent currently recommended. The target for NSP has already been mentioned above. Because of these targets, it is useful to know the amounts of different types of carbohydrate in foods. Examples are shown in Tables 1 and 2.

Table 2. Fibre (non-starch polysaccharide) content of selected foods (edible portion).

	Fibre (g/100 g)		Fibre (g/100 g)
Meat	0.0	Bread, white	1.5
Baked beans	3.7	Bread, brown	3.5
Beans, red kidney, boiled	6.7	Bread, wholemeal	5.8
Beans, runner, boiled	1.9	Flour, white	3.1
Cabbage, boiled	1.8	Flour, wholemeal	9.0
Carrots, boiled	2.5	All Bran	24.5
Potatoes, boiled	1.2	Porridge oats	7.1
Yams, boiled	1.4	Rice Krispies	0.7
Tomatoes, raw	1.0	Shredded wheat	9.8
Apples with skin, raw	1.8	Weetabix	9.7
Bananas	1.1	Rice, white, boiled	0.1
Raisins	2.0	Rice, brown, boiled	0.8
Nuts, mixed	6.0	Spaghetti, white, boiled	1.2
Biscuits, digestive	2.2	Spaghetti, wholemeal, boiled	3.5
Biscuits, rich tea	1.7		

The main sources of fibre in the diet are bread and other cereal products, vegetables and fruit.

Many individuals, particularly those of African, Asian and Indian races, have a limited ability to digest lactose. In later life some of these people may develop *lactose intolerance*, which results in digestive disturbances when the equivalent of a glass or more of milk is drunk. It is rarely found in healthy infants who depend on milk.

Diabetes is discussed on pp. 39 and 120.

3   Fats

Fats include not only 'visible fats' such as butter and margarine, cooking fats and oils and the fat on meat, but also the 'invisible fats' which occur in foods such as cheese, biscuits and cakes, nuts and other animal and vegetable foods. They are a more concentrated source of energy than carbohydrates, and are the form in which much of the energy reserve of animals and some seeds is stored.

Like carbohydrates, fats are compounds of carbon, hydrogen and oxygen only, but the proportion of oxygen is lower. Chemically, food fats consist mainly of mixtures of *triglycerides*. Each triglyceride is a combination of three *fatty acids* with a unit of glycerol (glycerine), and the differences between one fat or oil and another are largely the result of the different fatty acids in each.

Fatty acids

Many different fatty acids are found in nature. They differ in the number of carbon atoms they contain, and the number of hydrogen atoms held by the carbon atoms. *Saturated* fatty acids have as many hydrogen atoms as they can hold and this makes them stable so that they keep well. When hydrogen atoms are missing, carbon atoms form double bonds. *Monounsaturated* fatty acids contain only one double bond (two missing hydrogen atoms). *Polyunsaturated* fatty acids have two or more double bonds (four or more missing hydrogen atoms) which react gradually with oxygen in the air and make the fat rancid. All fats contain a mixture of these three types of fatty acid, but in widely varying proportions, depending on the source (Table 3 and Appendix 3). The presence of large amounts of unsaturated fatty acids in a mixture affects the physical as well as the chemical properties of a fat, making it liquid at room temperature (i.e. an oil). Some vegetable oils such as coconut and palm oils have a relatively high proportion of saturated fatty acids, but because these have a relatively low number of carbon atoms they do not cause the oil to solidify. In nature unsaturated fatty acids generally have their double bonds in the *cis* form. They can be changed into saturated fatty acids and a mixture of *cis* and *trans* monounsaturated fatty acids by controlled treatment with hydrogen (hydrogenation). This happens when liquid oils are hardened in the manufacture of margarine and cooking fats and, to a lesser extent, in the

Table 3. Average fatty acid composition of some foods, raw.

	Fat (g/100 g edible portion)	Fatty acids, per cent of fat by weight[a]		
		saturated	monounsaturated	polyunsaturated
Milk, cow's, whole	3.9	62	28	3
Milk, human	4.1	44	39	12
Cheese, Cheddar	34.4	63	27	4
Eggs	10.8	29	44	11
Beef, mince	16.2	43	48	4
Pork, chops	29.5	37	40	15
Chicken, light and dark meat	4.3	33	42	19
Liver, lamb's	10.3	28	29	15
Sardines, in tomato sauce	11.6	28	29	32
Butter	81.7	66	24	3
Margarine, hard	81.6	37	45	13
Margarine, soft	81.6	33	46	17
Margarine, polyunsaturated	81.6	20	25	50
Sunflower oil	99.9	12	20	63
Blended vegetable oil[b]	99.9	10	36	48
Potato crisps	37.6	24	32	26
Peanuts, roasted, salted	53.0	18	46	31
Biscuits, chocolate, fully coated	27.6	61	29	4
Chocolate, milk	30.3	59	31	5

[a] The total percentage of fatty acids is less than 100 because of the glycerol and other fatty compounds which are present. To calculate the total fatty acid content of a food, multiply the percentages of the various types of fatty acid by the amount of fat. Thus the total polyunsaturated fatty acid content of 100 g minced beef is $4/100 \times 16.2 = 0.65$ g.
[b] Average of several kinds; fatty acid profile of any one kind will depend on the particular blend of oils used in its manufacture.

rumen of cows and sheep. The more important fatty acids in foods are as follows:

SATURATED FATTY ACIDS

Palmitic acid and *stearic acid* are major constituents of hard fats such as butter, lard, suet and cocoa butter. *Myristic acid* occurs in butter and coconut oil.

Butyric acid, which, although present in only small amounts in milk fat and butter, makes an important contribution to their taste. Free butyric acid is released when these fats become rancid.

13

Oleic acid (monounsaturated) occurs in substantial amounts in all fats, but especially in olive oil and rapeseed oil where it provides 60–70 per cent of the total fatty acid content. *Trans* isomers of oleic and other monounsaturated fatty acids are found in hard margarines and shortenings and in products made from them such as biscuits and pastries, and in lesser amounts in ruminant fats (milk, cheese, beef and lamb).

Linoleic acid (with two double bonds) occurs in large amounts in vegetable seed oils such as maize (corn), soya bean and sunflower seed oils, and in small amounts in some animal fats such as pork.

Linolenic acid (with three double bonds, alpha form) occurs in small amounts in vegetable oils.

Arachidonic acid (with four double bonds) occurs in very small amounts in some animal fats. It can be formed in the body from linoleic acid.

A number of other polyunsaturated fatty acids occur in plants and fish oils, and are thought to be particularly beneficial to health. They include *gamma linolenic acid* (GLA), *docosahexaenoic acid* (DHA) and *eicosapentaenoic acid* (EPA). Polyunsaturated fatty acids can also be classified into *n-3* (omega-3) or *n-6* (omega-6) families, according to the position of the double bonds. DHA and EPA, which are obtained in the diet principally from oily fish, and alpha-linolenic acids belong to the *n-3* family. Linoleic, GLA and arachidonic acids belong to the *n-6* family and are obtained in the diet mainly from vegetable seeds and polyunsaturated margarines.

Both *n-3* and *n-6* polyunsaturated fatty acids must be present in the diet for normal health. Linoleic and alpha-linolenic acids are called 'essential fatty acids' because they cannot be made in the body. Arachidonic acid is sometimes regarded as essential if alpha-linolenic acid is in short supply. These fatty acids are required in small quantities in the diet for metabolism in the body to two families of *n-3* and *n-6* fatty acids which are necessary for the structure and functions of the tissues.

Properties of fats

Fats are solid at low temperatures and become liquid when they are heated. Oils are simply fats which are liquid at room temperature, usually as a result of their higher content of unsaturated fatty acids, and solidify on refrigeration (e.g. olive oil). Oils and fats do not dissolve in water, but may be *emulsified* with water by vigorous mixing as when butter, margarine and reduced-fat spreads are made. The oil and water usually separate again unless emulsifiers such as lecithin from soya beans or egg are added to the mixture.

Fats make an important contribution to food characteristics such as texture and palatability. Food fats usually contain small amounts of other fat-soluble substances, including flavour components and some of the vitamins. Animal fats may contain retinol (vitamin A) and vitamin D, and varying amounts of cholesterol, while vegetable fats may contain carotenes (which can be converted into vitamin A in the body) and vitamin E, but do not contain cholesterol.

The amount of energy obtained from a given weight of all common fats is about the same, despite the different functions and properties of many of the component fatty acids. It is more than double the energy, at 37 kJ per gram (9 kcal per gram), of an equal weight of carbohydrate or protein (see p. 30).

Mineral oils, such as liquid paraffin, are chemically different from food fats and oils despite their similarity in appearance. They cannot be utilised by the body, but function as laxatives and will reduce the absorption of some nutrients.

Sources of fat in the diet

VEGETABLE SOURCES

In plants, fats are formed from carbohydrate. Thus, when seeds such as sunflower and cottonseed ripen, their starch content decreases as their fat content rises. Oilseeds such as these and peanuts, coconuts, rapeseeds, palm kernels and soya beans contain about 20–40 per cent oil and are among the chief sources of oil for the manufacture of margarine and cooking fat. The fat content of flour and other cereal products (apart from oatmeal) is generally low, as is the fat content of most vegetables and fruits. The proportion of each fatty acid present varies from plant to plant, and is also quite variable within a species. Vegetable seeds are among the principal sources of *n-6* polyunsaturated fatty acids.

ANIMAL SOURCES

Animals, including humans, store excess energy almost entirely in deposits of fat, the amount of which is very variable. As in plants, this fat can be made from carbohydrate – but the dietary carbohydrate can be starch, sugar or even (in cows and sheep) cellulose. Animals also lay down fat from their dietary fat; in this case the fatty acid composition reflects that of the diet, except for ruminants whose digestive processes normally make the fatty acids more saturated.

Fish such as herring, mackerel, pilchards, salmon, sardines, tuna and eels are sometimes called *oily fish*. The proportion of fat in them varies with the season of the year. Fish oils are the principal sources of *n-3* polyunsaturated fatty acids. *White fish* such as cod, haddock and plaice contain little fat except in the liver. Fish liver is also a rich source of vitamins A and D.

The fat content of many foods, especially meat, varies widely. Average values, and the main sources of fat in the British diet, are shown in Table 4.

Table 4. Average fat content of foods, raw (edible portion).

	Fat (g/100 g)		Fat (g/100 g)
Milk, whole	3.9	Cod, filleted	0.7
Milk, semi-skimmed	1.6	Mackerel	16.3
Milk, skimmed	0.1	Tuna, canned in oil, drained	9.0
Yogurt, low fat, fruit	0.7	Butter	81.7
Ice cream, non-dairy	8.7	Margarine	81.6
Cheese, Cheddar	34.4	Low-fat spread	40.5
Cheese, Edam	25.4	Very-low-fat spread	25.0
Cheese, cottage	3.9	Vegetable oils	99.9
Eggs	10.8	Lard and dripping	99.0
Beef, stewing steak	10.6	Potatoes, old	0.2
Lamb, leg	18.7	Chips, fried, take-away	12.4
Pork, chop	29.5	Chips, oven-baked	4.2
Bacon, streaky	39.5	Peanut butter	53.7
Sausages, pork	32.1	Bread, white	1.9
Beefburgers	20.5	Bread, wholemeal	2.5
Chicken, meat and skin	17.7	Porridge oats	9.2
Turkey, meat and skin	6.9	Biscuits, digestive	20.9

The main sources of fat in the diet are fats and oils including margarine, butter and low-fat spreads, meat and meat products, cakes and biscuits, and whole milk.

Throughout the world the amount of fat in the diet tends to be higher in affluent than in poor countries, and within poorer countries, higher in the wealthier families. Less than 10 per cent of the energy value of the diet is derived from fat in many of the world's poorest countries. In most developed countries, including Britain, fat has for many years provided about 40 per cent of energy. In Britain this proportion is very similar across all income groups.

The amount of dietary energy derived from saturated fatty acids has been falling and the average proportion of polyunsaturated to saturated fatty acids (the 'P/S ratio') in the whole diet is about 0.4:1, having risen from about 0.2:1 in 1970.

Health aspects of fats

Diets in poor countries are often low in energy, and the World Health Organization (WHO) has recommended an increase in fat intakes in such situations. Conversely there is a need to decrease the fat content of the diets of affluent populations as a means of reducing the risk of various diseases, notably heart disease but also, possibly, some types of cancer.

To ensure that sufficient quantities of essential fatty acids are present in our diets, COMA (see p. 8) recommends that linoleic and alpha-linolenic acids, which were once called vitamin F, should provide at least 1 and 0.2 per cent, respectively, of the total dietary energy. At the same time, to encourage a decrease in total fat and saturated fatty acid intake, average values have been set for the UK population which are advisable to achieve in terms of the proportion of dietary energy to be consumed as different types of fatty acids (see below).

HEART DISEASE

In the UK, in both men and women, *coronary heart disease* (CHD) is a serious health problem. The risk of heart disease is increased by various factors such as smoking, high blood pressure and raised levels of cholesterol in the blood. All, except smoking, are influenced by the diet. Obesity can affect both blood pressure and blood cholesterol and is discussed on p. 28. Blood pressure can also be increased by excessive intakes of alcohol (see p. 101) and by obesity. It may also be raised in certain people by high intakes of sodium. High saturated fatty acid intakes can lead to increased blood cholesterol levels, particularly in susceptible individuals.

Cholesterol is mostly made in the liver and is carried in the blood mainly by two proteins – *low-density lipoprotein* (LDL) and *high-density lipoprotein* (HDL). LDL cholesterol is considered to be undesirable because if it increases to a high level in the blood it can be deposited on the walls of the blood vessels thereby helping to form 'plaques' that may eventually lead to narrowing of the arteries which supply the heart with blood. This is more likely to happen if the LDL is modified chemically by oxidation (p. 66). If the arteries become blocked completely with further plaque or by a blood clot, the blood supply to the heart is interrupted leading to a heart attack and, in severe cases, to death. HDL cholesterol is desirable as it is a means of transporting cholesterol from parts of the body where there is too much to the liver where it can be disposed of. Replacing saturated by monounsaturated or polyunsaturated fatty acids in the diet can lower LDL blood cholesterol. The cholesterol in food has a smaller effect on blood cholesterol than do saturated fatty acids, but the effect varies in different people. The liver can compensate for changes in dietary cholesterol by changing the amount of cholesterol it makes.

The *n-3* polyunsaturated fatty acids in fish oils do not seem to have a major effect on blood cholesterol levels, but may help to prevent heart disease by decreasing the tendency of the blood to clot and keeping the heart cell membranes stable. Current recommendations are that the average intake of *n-3* polyunsaturated fatty acids for the population should double to about 0.2 g per day (1.5 g per week). This would be achieved by increasing consumption of oily fish.

The Government advises that the population average intakes of fat and saturated fatty acids should reduce to the levels recommended in 1991 (see Table 26, Chapter 9) in order to help achieve a decrease in heart disease.

A review of the nutritional aspects of heart disease in 1994 made further recommendations on fat intakes that were substantially the same as those made in 1991: on average, total fat and saturated fatty acids should provide not more than about 35 per cent and 10 per cent, respectively, of dietary energy intake; n-6 polyunsaturated fatty acids should continue to provide about 6 per cent of energy; and the average intake of dietary cholesterol should not increase. Between 1986 and 1997, fat and saturated fatty acid contributions to food energy intake fell from about 43 to 39 per cent and about 18 to 15 per cent, respectively. Many people therefore still need to be encouraged to make substantial changes to their diets if the average fat intake of the population is to decrease to the desired level.

Trans fatty acids may have undesirable effects on blood LDL and HDL cholesterol and may increase the risk of coronary heart disease. The present average intake of *trans* fatty acids in Britain is about 5 g per day or 2 per cent of food energy. Current recommendations are that *trans* fatty acids should provide no more than 2 per cent of dietary energy and that ways of decreasing the average amount in people's diets should be considered.

CANCER

In a report published in 1998, the Committee on Medical Aspects of Food and Nutrition Policy (COMA) concluded that there was not sufficiently strong evidence linking total fat intakes to the development of cancers to make any specific recommendations. The report's recommendations include maintenance of a healthy body weight, and increased intakes of a variety of fruit and vegetables and of fibre from a variety of food sources. For adults, it also recommends that individuals' intake of red and processed meat should not increase and that high consumers of these foods should consider a reduction. As a guide, average UK intakes are about 90 g per day and high intakes above 140 g per day (both on a cooked weight basis). These recommendations are made in the light of existing COMA recommendations including those to reduce the average fat intake of the populations (see page 71).

4 Proteins

All proteins are compounds of carbon, hydrogen and oxygen, but unlike carbohydrates and fats, they always contain nitrogen as well. Most proteins also contain sulphur (present in only a few amino acids) and some contain phosphorus. They are essential constituents of all cells, where they regulate the processes of life or provide structure. Protein must be provided in the diet for the growth and repair of the body, but any excess is used to provide energy.

Proteins consist of chains of hundreds or even thousands of *amino acid* units. Only about 20 different amino acids are used, but the number of ways in which they can be arranged is almost infinite. It is the specific and unique sequence of these units which gives each protein its characteristic structural and enzymatic properties.

Amino acids

It is convenient to divide amino acids into two types: *indispensable* and *dispensable*. *Indispensable* amino acids cannot be made in the body, at least in amounts sufficient for health, and must therefore be present in the food. *Dispensable* amino acids are equally necessary as components of all proteins in the body; they differ only in that it is possible for them to be made from any excess of certain other amino acids in the diet. The eight amino acids indispensable for *adults* are:

Isoleucine	Phenylalanine
Leucine	Threonine
Lysine	Tryptophan
Methionine	Valine

A further amino acid, histidine, is also indispensable for the rapidly growing *infant*. The remaining amino acids which are found in proteins are:

Alanine	Glutamine
Arginine	Glycine
Aspartic acid	Proline
Asparagine	Serine
Cysteine	Tyrosine
Glutamic acid	

Animal and vegetable proteins

The overall proportions of amino acids in any single vegetable food (cereals, nuts and seeds, potatoes, or legumes such as peas and beans) differ from those needed by humans. For example, wheat and rice proteins are comparatively low in lysine, and legumes such as lentils are low in tryptophan and methionine (Table 5). These proteins are therefore said to have low *biological values*, because the *quality* of a protein depends on its ability to supply all the indispensable amino acids in the amounts needed. Mixtures of such foods, however, complement each other and result in greatly enhanced values so that, even among those who eat little or no animal protein, deficiency is rarely a problem provided they have enough food to eat.

Most animal proteins (from meat, fish, milk, cheese and eggs) have a high biological value. The reason for this is that humans are part of the animal kingdom; the proteins of animals are therefore more like ours and can be utilised by us with the minimum of waste. In effect, animals have pre-selected, with varying degrees of efficiency, the plant amino acids which they and we

Table 5. **Proportion of some indispensable amino acids in selected proteins.**

	Amino acid content (g/100 g protein)		
	Lysine	Methionine	Tryptophan
Milk, cow's	8.4	2.9	1.5
Eggs	6.2	3.1	1.8
Beef	9.1	2.7	1.3
Fish, cod	9.8	2.9	1.1
Lentils	6.7	0.7	0.9
Peanuts	4.0	1.3	1.3
Wheat flour[a]	2.7	1.8	1.3
Rice[a]	3.3	1.8	1.2

[a] Some amino acids can be increased by genetic breeding.

need and have burned up the remainder for energy (p. 39). Nevertheless, the nutritional advantages of animal foods over vegetable foods in practice lie more in the presence of associated nutrients such as vitamin B_{12}, iron and retinol (pre-formed vitamin A) than in the protein.

Because there is no way in which excesses of amino acids can be stored in the body, they will be most efficiently used if a complete assortment is supplied to the body at about the same time. This can be achieved by eating a mixed diet at each meal and ensuring that the total energy content of the diet is also adequate. Mixtures of vegetable protein foods such as beans on toast, or of animal and vegetable foods such as fish and chips, bread and cheese, and breakfast cereals with milk, therefore have a sound physiological basis.

Novel sources of protein

Animals convert plant protein into their own muscle slowly and inefficiently (only 5–10 per cent being retained). There is a growing demand for sources of protein which are suitable for vegetarians. Some people may also want to limit their fat intake and eat protein-rich foods which do not contain fat. As a response to these factors, products providing alternatives to meat have been developed by the food industry. In addition to those described below, soya-based foods such as tofu (bean curd) and miso (fermented bean paste), which are traditionally used in Far Eastern cuisine, are now increasingly available in the UK.

Texturised vegetable proteins have been developed by concentrating or isolating the proteins from a number of plants, especially soya beans, and converting them directly into products such as soya 'mince' or soya 'chunks'. If suitably fortified with the most important minerals and vitamins which meat provides, such as thiamin, riboflavin, vitamin B_{12}, iron and zinc, these products can be used instead of meat and are acceptable to vegetarians (vegetarian diets are discussed on p. 119).

Mycoprotein is another product which can be used as an alternative to meat. One type, made from a particular fungal microorganism and complying with a particular specification, has been cleared for human consumption. It is manufactured commercially (Quorn) and is produced by growing the fungal microorganism in a fermenter and 'harvesting' the product. This is heat-processed, seasoned and cooked, and then sliced, diced or shredded. It can be used instead of meat in home recipes and is also incorporated into a range of retailed products, for example pies and recipe dishes.

It is also possible to utilise other microorganisms such as yeast, or otherwise inedible leaves, to provide protein-rich foods for animals and humans.

Protein as a source of energy

The amount and type of protein in the diet will not exactly balance the requirements for growth, repair and maintenance: there will always be excesses of some amino acids, and usually an excess of total protein. These will be converted into glucose in the liver or be directly oxidised to provide heat and energy. Furthermore, if the energy available from the diet is insufficient to meet demands, this oxidation of the amino acids tends to take preference over their more fundamental use for rebuilding proteins. This is why it is important to ensure that diets contain sufficient energy in the form of carbohydrate and fat before proteins are added, for only then can these proteins be properly utilised for purposes which no other nutrient can fulfil.

Other health aspects of proteins

Newborn infants can absorb some proteins intact from their mothers' milk, including antibodies which provide protection from infection. Susceptible individuals can also react adversely to certain food proteins: for example, those with coeliac disease react to gluten and others may react to cow's milk protein and nut proteins, in rare cases with fatal results.

Certain beans including red kidney beans and soya beans contain proteins which are harmful, unless thoroughly cooked in *moist* heat such as boiling water.

Properties of proteins

Some proteins dissolve in water and some in salt water. Some are insoluble and this is exploited in the preparation of wheat gluten, which is used to improve the baking quality of home-produced wheats, by washing other proteins and starch from a wheat dough. The separated starch is used for producing glucose syrups.

The action of heat on proteins is complex. Proteins such as the albumen in egg white harden or coagulate irreversibly when heated, but are still readily digested. Individual amino acids are little affected by normal cooking procedures, although some of the lysine may react with carbohydrates in the food (e.g. in the baking of bread) and methionine may sometimes be reduced. In the preparation of gelatin, however, when connective tissue from meat is boiled for many hours, *all* the tryptophan is destroyed.

Complex reactions between amino acids (usually lysine) and sugars in foods (the Maillard reaction) result in the attractive golden brown colour of crisps or chips and also in the formation of certain desirable food flavours. However, they may also give rise to the brown discoloration which sometimes develops during prolonged storage of concentrated or dried milk or dehydrated vegetables.

Sources of protein in the diet

About one-third of the protein in the average UK diet comes from plant sources and two-thirds from animal sources. The amount of protein in nuts and dried peas and beans is very high – about the same as in meat, fish and cheese. The proportion is reduced when these pulses are soaked in water, but they remain an excellent source of protein. Cereals are also rich in protein; indeed wheat, maize and rice are the main sources of protein for many people in the world. The amount of protein in roots and tubers is small, but as potatoes are eaten in quantity they provide useful amounts. Many green and leafy vegetables contain some protein, but because they are often eaten in small amounts or infrequently by some sectors of the UK population they make little contribution to average protein intakes. The concentration of protein in selected foods is shown in Table 6.

Table 6. Average protein content of selected foods, uncooked.

	Protein (g/100 g)		Protein (g/100 g)
Milk, cow's, whole	3.2	Baked beans	5.2
Milk, cow's, skimmed	3.3	Beans, red kidney, dry	22.1
Soya drink (previously called		Soya tofu, steamed	8.1
soya milk)	2.9	Peanuts	25.6
Cheese, Cheddar	25.5	Peas, frozen	6.0
Cheese, feta	15.6	Sweetcorn, canned	2.9
Beef, stewing	20.2	Potatoes	2.1
Lamb, leg	17.9	Apples	0.4
Pork, chop	15.9	Bread, white	8.4
Sausages, pork	10.6	Bread, wholemeal	9.2
Chicken	17.6	Flour, white	9.4
Turkey	20.6	Cornflakes	7.9
Cod	17.4	Mycoprotein	11.8
Prawns	22.6	Spaghetti, dry	12.0

The main sources of protein in the diet are meat, milk, bread and other cereals.

5 Energy needs and food consumption

Uses of energy

Energy, which gives us the ability to do work, is obtained from food by controlled oxidation of the carbohydrates, fat, protein and alcohol in the diet. It is necessary for three purposes:

(a) to maintain life
(b) for muscular activity, and
(c) for additional needs during growth, pregnancy and lactation.

If more is obtained than is used in these ways, the excess is stored in the body as fat.

MAINTENANCE OF LIFE

Energy is required for breathing, the heartbeat, the maintenance of body temperature, and other involuntary activities including brain function. The amount needed can be measured in people at complete rest or asleep. This *basal metabolic rate* (BMR) is higher in relation to body size in infants and actively growing young children than in adults. After adolescence, the needs are proportional to the amount of lean tissue in the body; thus women tend to have lower resting metabolic rates than men both because they are lighter and because muscle generally forms a lower proportion of their body weight (and fat a higher proportion). The BMR is also lower in elderly people, or during starvation, because of the reduction which occurs in lean tissue. It is thus possible to adapt to changed energy intakes.

After food is eaten, extra heat is produced and more energy is needed to cover this. The amount varies with the food. Climate does not significantly affect the resting metabolism, but the rate does vary widely between apparently similar individuals because the efficiency of the body processes varies. Average values of the BMR for the two sexes in different age groups can be estimated from body weight using suitable equations (see Appendix 2).

Some examples are:

	Weight (kg)	Basal metabolic rate (BMR) (resting energy requirement)	
		MJ(kcal)/day	MJ (kcal)/kg/day
Infant, 1 year old	10	2.3 (560)	0.23 (56)
Boy, 10 years old	33	5.2 (1240)	0.16 (38)
Man, 40 years old	76	7.3 (1750)	0.10 (23)
Woman, 40 years old	62	5.7 (1360)	0.09 (22)
Man, 75+ years old	69	5.8 (1400)	0.08 (20)

A man therefore needs about 5 kJ (a little more than 1 kcal) each minute just to keep alive. During 8 hours sleep, the resting requirement of about 2.4 MJ (580 kcal) is all that would be used, but during the remainder of the day the additional requirements of physical activity must be taken into account.

ACTIVITY

Whenever people move, they use extra energy. The heavier they are the more it takes, and strenuous activities require more energy than light ones. There are also substantial variations between apparently similar individuals. Measuring the energy cost of different activities for people with different body weights is very time consuming. Instead the energy used for a particular physical activity can be calculated by multiplying the BMR by a factor appropriate to that activity. This factor, the *physical activity ratio* (PAR), is calculated as follows:

$$PAR = \frac{\text{the energy cost of an activity per minute}}{\text{the energy cost of the BMR per minute}}$$

Thus the energy cost for sitting at rest is $1.2 \times$ BMR; for walking at a normal pace $4 \times$ BMR; for jogging $7 \times$ BMR, etc. By combining all these activities over a 24-hour period, a multiple of the BMR which characterises a person's lifestyle can be derived. This multiple – the *physical activity level* (PAL) – is calculated as follows:

$$PAL = \frac{\text{the total energy required over 24 hours}}{\text{the BMR over 24 hours}}$$

Daily energy expenditure can be estimated by multiplying BMR by PAL. A PAL of 1.4, representing very little physical activity at work or during leisure time, applies to most people in the UK. Values for PAL of 1.6 for women and 1.7 for men represent moderate activity during work time and leisure; PAL values of 1.8 for women and 1.9 for men represent high levels of activity at work and during recreation.

Some examples of the energy expended on activities by an average 25-year-old woman office worker weighing 62 kg (10 stone) are shown below:

	Average energy expenditure	
	(kJ/min)	(kcal/min)
Everyday activities		
Sitting, eating	5	1.1
Standing, cooking	9	2.1
Washing and dressing	9	2.1
Walking moderately quickly	15	3.5
Walking up and down stairs	28	6.5
Work and recreation		
Office, sitting	6	1.5
Office, walking slowly	11	2.6
Dancing	19	4.5
Average jogging	27	6.5

Total energy requirements

The dietary energy required by an individual who is neither gaining nor losing weight exactly equals the energy expended on maintenance and physical activity. In practice this balance is achieved over periods of a few days, with remarkable accuracy: an excessive intake of only 40 kJ (10 kcal) each day would be equivalent to a weight gain of about 0.5 kg (1 lb) every year. The energy expended during a day can be estimated from the BMR and the average PAR values for various activities, taking into account the time spent on each. A male sedentary worker, such as a civil servant, with a moderately active leisure time, might expend 10.9 MJ (2633 kcal) in a typical day as shown at the top of the next page.

The example used is of a man 40 years old, weighing 76 kg and having a BMR of 7.3 MJ per day. His physical activity level (PAL) would be 1.5 (Total energy expenditure divided by BMR). Because of individual variations, the diet of any particular sedentary worker may provide more or less energy than this; the average intake of a group of such people would, however, be expected to be close to this value. In summary, the daily energy requirement of any adult is that amount which maintains the desirable body weight.

BODY SIZE AND COMPOSITION

Heavy people use more energy for maintenance and physical activity, although some may spend less time than lighter people in activities. Women tend to need less energy than men, although their needs are increased during the last months of pregnancy and during lactation.

26

	PAR	Average energy expenditure	
		(MJ)	(kcal)
8 h asleep	1.0	2.4	576
8 h at work			
6½ h sitting	1.4	2.7	652
1½ h standing and slow walking	1.8	0.8	194
8 h non-occupational activities			
15 min washing and dressing	2.5	0.2	45
2 h 15 min commuting	1.7	1.1	273
1½ h light domestic chores	2.2	1.0	273
3 h sitting, eating, reading, watching TV	1.2	1.1	258
30 min squash	7.5	1.1	273
30 min light gardening	3.5	0.5	125
Total energy expenditure (TEE)		10.9	2633

AGE

Requirements for maintenance are proportionately highest in infants and young children, and usually lowest in elderly people who have less lean body tissue and are less active.

PHYSICAL ACTIVITY

The degree of activity is the most important factor in determining energy requirements, and also the most difficult to assess. Sedentary workers (for example, those who spend most of their time at an office desk or behind the wheel of a motor vehicle) need a total of about 3.8 MJ (900 kcal) for 8 hours work; moderately active people (many industrial workers, nursing staff and postal workers) need about 5.0 MJ (1200 kcal), and very active workers (oil rig workers, building labourers, farm workers, fishing crews and armed forces recruits) have an average need for about 7.5 MJ (1800 kcal) during 8 hours at work. Leisure activities such as jogging, particularly if indulged in regularly or for long periods, also affect the day's requirements.

GROWTH, PREGNANCY AND LACTATION

Additional energy is needed during growth to provide for the extra body tissue. In newborn infants, about one-third of the total energy needs is used for laying down new tissue. However, this falls to about 4 per cent of total energy needs by one year of age and even in the rapidly growing child this need remains small in comparison with the requirement for maintenance and movement.

During pregnancy and lactation (breastfeeding), all the infant's needs for energy (as for other nutrients, see p. 114) must be supplied by the mother. Extra food energy is needed during the final months of pregnancy (0.8 MJ (200 kcal) per day during the last trimester). Some of this is used to build up a store of about 2 kg of fat in the mother, which may be gradually drawn upon during lactation, but an additional intake of 1.9–2.4 MJ (450–570 kcal) per day from the diet is also recommended from the start of lactation to three months onwards (p. 116).

Obesity

When a person has an excessive amount of body fat they are said to be obese. Of British adults surveyed in 1991, a high proportion (13 per cent of men and 15 per cent of women) were obese. Such people have a greater risk of developing diseases which include diabetes, cardiovascular disease, high blood pressure and some cancers.

If individuals eat or drink foods which provide more energy than they use up in their daily activities, some of the fat, protein, carbohydrate or alcohol will be converted into body fat, the most readily convertible nutrient being fat. Any kind of food can therefore be 'fattening' if eaten in sufficient quantity. Some foods, however, are more concentrated sources of energy than others. These tend to be foods containing little water and a high proportion of fat, such as butter, margarine, fatty meat, fried foods, ice cream, cakes and biscuits. High palatability of foods can also encourage excessive amounts to be eaten. Obesity may occur even if energy intake is only slightly greater than output if it is consistently so over a long period of time.

The broad range of weights found for people at different heights has been used to construct the chart shown in Figure 1. This can be used to indicate whether an individual is an acceptable weight for their height. The *Body Mass Index* (BMI), calculated as weight in kilograms divided by the square of the height in metres, is also used to assess the degree to which a person is overweight. A BMI of below 20 is underweight; 20–24 is desirable; 25–30 is overweight; and above 30 is considered obese.

Weight may be lost by decreasing energy intake or increasing physical activity or both. Conversely, weight may be gained by increasing energy intake, or decreasing physical activity. The exact consequences of these changes are difficult to predict because of the large differences between individual responses and some measure of adaptation, but for many people the part played by changes in activity may be comparatively small. For example, if a man trying to lose weight takes a brisk half-hour walk, he will expend about 420 kJ (100 kcal) more than if he sat watching television. If at the end of his walk, however, he is thirsty and drinks a pint of beer, he will take in substantially more energy than he used up. If this happens frequently he

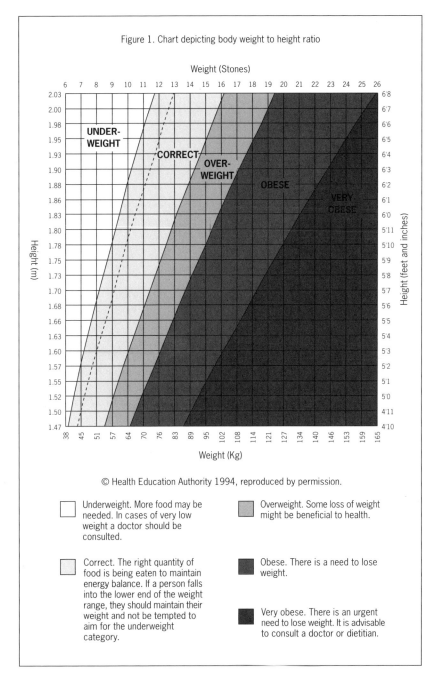

Figure 1. Chart depicting body weight to height ratio

© Health Education Authority 1994, reproduced by permission.

☐ Underweight. More food may be needed. In cases of very low weight a doctor should be consulted.

☐ Correct. The right quantity of food is being eaten to maintain energy balance. If a person falls into the lower end of the weight range, they should maintain their weight and not be tempted to aim for the underweight category.

▨ Overweight. Some loss of weight might be beneficial to health.

■ Obese. There is a need to lose weight.

■ Very obese. There is an urgent need to lose weight. It is advisable to consult a doctor or dietitian.

29

should not be surprised if his weight increases. Nevertheless, *regular* vigorous exercise can be an important factor in weight control.

Eating disorders

It is important to realise that some body fat is essential for health, but some people, particularly teenage girls, seek to reduce their weight below the desirable range shown in Figure 1. *Anorexia nervosa* and *bulimia nervosa* are psychological conditions expressed by extremes of behaviour involving food avoidance or alternate binge-eating and vomiting, respectively, and can be fatal.

Energy value of food

The energy provided by the fat, protein and carbohydrate in food, and by alcohol, can be measured. Taking into account the small proportions of these macronutrients which are not absorbed into the body, it is accepted that:

1 g dietary carbohydrate (calculated as monosaccharides) provides 16 kJ or 3.75 kcal
1 g dietary fat provides 37 kJ or 9 kcal
1 g dietary protein provides 17 kJ or 4 kcal
1 g alcohol provides 29 kJ or 7 kcal.

Polyols also provide energy (see p. 6) and small amounts of energy can be derived from organic acids such as citric acid in fruits and drinks and acetic acid in vinegar, with each gram providing approximately 13 kJ (3 kcal). The micronutrients (minerals and vitamins), fibre and water do not provide energy.

The energy value of any food can be calculated when the proportions of the nutrients in it are known. For example, if 100 g of potato crisps contain 49.3 g carbohydrate, 37.6 g fat and 5.6 g protein, the energy content is calculated as follows:

$$
\begin{array}{lll}
49.3 \times 16 & = & 788.8 \text{ kJ from carbohydrate} \\
37.6 \times 37 & = & 1391.2 \text{ kJ from fat} \\
5.6 \times 17 & = & 95.2 \text{ kJ from protein} \\
\text{Total} & & 2275.2 \text{ kJ}
\end{array}
$$

or

$$
\begin{array}{lll}
49.3 \times 3.75 & = & 184.9 \text{ kcal from carbohydrate} \\
37.6 \times 9 & = & 338.4 \text{ kcal from fat} \\
5.6 \times 4 & = & 22.4 \text{ kcal from protein} \\
\text{Total} & & 545.7 \text{ kcal}
\end{array}
$$

It is misleading, however, to imply that energy values can be obtained with such precision; decimal points should not be included in the results, which might be rounded to 2275 kJ or 546 kcal. But when performing further calculations such as for the proportion of energy derived from fat, it is wiser to use the detailed figures and round off only at the end (see also Appendix 4):

$$\frac{1391.2}{2275.2} \times 100 = 61.15 \text{ or } 61 \text{ per cent of energy from fat}$$

Sources of energy in the diet

Nearly all the weight of any food is made up of protein, fat and carbohydrate together with water. Foods which contain large amounts of water, such as salad vegetables, fruit and clear soups will contain little protein, fat or carbohydrate, and consequently provide little energy. In contrast, dry foods such as breakfast cereals, and foods rich in fat (each gram of which provides more than twice as much energy as each gram of protein or carbohydrate) and in sugar are concentrated sources of energy. The main sources of energy in the UK diet are bread, flour and other cereals, meat, visible fats, dairy produce and sugar – foods which are not only rich in energy but also eaten in substantial quantities. For some people, sweets and alcoholic drinks are also a significant source of energy. The energy (and water) contents of selected foods are shown in Table 7.

The significance of hot foods

The energy provided by the heat of hot food is trifling compared with the energy provided by metabolism of its constituents within the body. For example, the constituents of cream of tomato soup provide 230 kJ (55 kcal) per 100 g; a serving of 250 ml (250 g or 9 oz) would therefore provide about 580 kJ (140 kcal). The additional heat provided by its cooling from a serving temperature of, say 60°C to the body temperature of 37°C would be about 25 kJ (6 kcal). Nevertheless, this heat is immediately perceived, and can give a useful boost to morale on cold days.

Table 7. Average energy value and water content of selected foods (edible portion).

	Energy		Water (g/100 g)
	(kJ/100 g)	(kcal/100 g)	
Milk, whole	275	66	88
Milk, semi-skimmed	195	46	90
Milk, skimmed	140	33	90
Cheese, Cheddar	1708	412	36
Yogurt, low-fat, fruit	382	90	77
Beef, stewing steak (lean and fat), stewed	932	223	57
Bacon, streaky (lean and fat), fried	2050	496	27
Chicken, roast, meat only	621	148	68
Cod, fillet, baked	408	96	77
Fish fingers, grilled	899	214	56
Sardines, canned in oil, drained	906	217	58
Eggs, boiled	612	147	75
Butter/margarine	3035	738	16
Low-fat spread	1605	390	50
Vegetable oil	8696	899	0
Sugar	1680	394	0
Courgettes, boiled	81	19	93
Lettuce	59	14	95
Carrots, old, boiled	100	24	91
Potatoes, old, boiled	306	72	80
Chips, fried in blended oil, take-away	1001	239	52
Apples	199	47	85
Banana, flesh only	403	95	75
Sultanas	1171	275	15
Orange, flesh only	158	37	86
Bread, white	1002	235	37
Bread, wholemeal	914	215	38
Biscuits, chocolate, full coated	2197	524	2
Cornflakes	1535	360	3
Crispbread, rye	1367	321	6
Lager	120	29	95
Wine, white, medium	311	75	86
Spirits	919	222	63

6 Digestion of food and absorption of major nutrients

Food has been defined as any solid or liquid which, when swallowed, can provide the body with energy, or material for growth and repair, or certain substances for regulating body processes. However, it is clear that almost any food can be recovered virtually intact from the stomach if vomiting occurs soon after it is eaten. Therefore, food cannot really be said to have entered the body until it has been:

(a) *digested*, i.e. physically and chemically broken down into simple component parts which can be

(b) *absorbed*, i.e. passed through the walls of the digestive tract into the blood (or lymph)

Flavour and appetite

For food to be eaten, it must be appetizing or we must be hungry – preferably both circumstances should apply. When and how much we eat is determined by a number of factors.

The complex sensation of *hunger* occurs when the body's stores are reduced (giving rise to reduced levels of glucose and fatty acids in the blood) and the stomach is empty. But people, especially obese people, do not eat only when they are hungry and stop when they cease to feel hungry. *Appetite* is a sensation which relates to the smell and taste of particular foods and their ingredients, and is influenced by the surroundings, habits and emotional state of the individual, all of which can also increase or decrease the flow of saliva and other digestive juices. Thus, where there is freedom of choice, more attractive foods are likely to be eaten in preference to others, and it can be seen that good cooking and pleasant surroundings are important in nutrition. It should, however, be noted that some appetizing foods such as confectionery products can be relatively low in many nutrients, and that unappetizing foods can provide nourishment – as when an unconscious person is fed through a naso-gastric tube.

The process of digestion

Although cooking softens meat fibres and the cellulose of plant materials, and gelatinises starch, true digestion only begins when food enters the mouth and

33

digestive tract. The digestive tract, illustrated in Figure 2, is basically a tube about 5 m long.

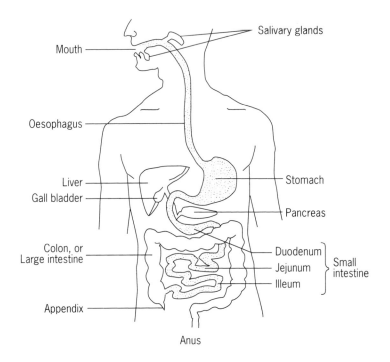

Figure 2. Diagram of digestive system

IN THE MOUTH

(a) Food is mechanically broken down by chewing. It is therefore important to have healthy teeth and gums.
(b) The food is mixed and moistened with saliva.

Saliva comes from salivary glands under the tongue and at the back of the mouth. It is usually present in the mouth, but its flow is increased by the smell and taste of food and by chewing. It helps the food to be swallowed, and also contains an enzyme, salivary *amylase*, which converts a small amount of the starch into maltose.

After the mixture of food particles and saliva has been swallowed – the final voluntary action – it takes about 3 seconds to pass down the oesophagus into the stomach, where:
(a) the food is mixed with gastric juice
(b) more mechanical breakdown results from stomach contractions.

Gastric juice is produced by the lining of the stomach in response to the same stimuli that increase saliva flow. Normally, about 3 litres are produced each day. It has three important constituents:
(a) the enzyme *pepsin*, which begins the digestion of protein
(b) about 0.2 to 0.4 per cent of hydrochloric acid (much more acid than in 'acid foods') that destroys most of the bacteria which could be present in food and water and provides the acid conditions necessary for the pepsin to be active.
(c) 'Intrinsic factor', necessary for subsequent absorption of vitamin B_{12}.

Speed of digestion in the stomach

The main function of the stomach is to act as a reservoir: digestion still proceeds if the stomach is completely removed. Food normally remains there for 2 to 4 hours before the resulting semi-liquid mixture (chyme) is passed by degrees into the small intestine. The exact time depends on the emotional state of the person and the type of food eaten: foods rich in carbohydrate (such as rice) pass most quickly and those rich in fat most slowly.

Despite its name, the small intestine is the longest part of the digestive tract. It is about 3 m in length (although because of the loss of tone and elasticity, it is found to be 7–8 m long after death), compared with about 1 m for the large intestine. It is, however, only 2–4 cm in diameter compared with 6 cm for the latter. The first distinct part of the small intestine is called the *duodenum*; the remainder consists of the *jejunum* and finally the *ileum*. It is in this organ that the main part of both digestion and absorption takes place.

In the duodenum, the digestive juices poured on to the food mixture from three sources are:
(a) *bile*, which is produced in the liver and stored in the gall bladder. Bile salts emulsify the fat into microscopic droplets so that it can be digested.
(b) *pancreatic juice*, from the pancreas. This alkaline liquid neutralizes the acid chyme, and contains a number of enzymes for breaking down fats, proteins and carbohydrates into their component parts. The most important of these are *lipase* which splits fatty acids from triglycerides of fat, *trypsin* and *chymotrypsin* which split proteins into small peptides and amino acids, and *amylase* which splits starch into maltose.

(c) *intestinal juice*, from the walls of the small intestine itself. This also contains digestive enzymes.

The final phase of digestion occurs *in* the intestinal wall after absorption, when peptides are split into their component amino acids, maltose is converted into glucose by *maltase*, sucrose into glucose and fructose by *sucrase*, and lactose into glucose and galactose by *lactase*. A summary of the major enzymes of digestion is provided in Table 8.

Table 8. Summary of the major enzymes of digestion.

Enzyme	Where active	Action
Salivary amylase	Mouth	Some starch to maltose
Pepsin	Stomach	Protein to peptides
Rennin (in infants only)	Stomach	Milk protein to peptides
Trypsin (from pancreas)	Intestine	Protein to peptides and amino acids
Chymotrypsin (from pancreas)	Intestine	Protein to peptides and amino acids
Lipase (from pancreas and intestine)	Intestine	Fat to fatty acids
Amylase (from pancreas)	Intestine	Starch (and glycogen) to maltose
Maltase	Intestinal wall	Maltose to glucose
Sucrase	Intestinal wall	Sucrose to glucose and fructose
Lactase	Intestinal wall	Lactose to glucose and galactose

IN THE LARGE INTESTINE

Substances which have resisted digestion and absorption thus far can be used for food by the bacteria present in the large intestine (colon). Some cellulose and other components of fibre may then be broken down, and the bacteria will form B-vitamins and vitamin K which provide small amounts of additional nutrients for absorption. They also generate gas (mainly hydrogen).

DIGESTION IN INFANTS

Before birth, infants are nourished through their bloodstream via the mother's placenta. The change to intestinal digestion does not develop fully for several months after birth. Three consequences in particular may be noted:

(a) for a few days, some whole proteins can be absorbed without digestion. In this way, antibodies against some diseases may be absorbed intact from the mother's milk.

(b) the stomach contains the enzyme *rennin*, which clots the casein of milk and begins its digestion.

(c) starch cannot readily be digested until the infant is several months old.

36

A food or food component is indigestible if it cannot be fully broken down into substances capable of absorption. Some, such as lactose from milk in lactose-intolerant individuals, will reach the large intestine and be fermented by the bacteria present; this results in the production of gas and diarrhoea. Indigestion also means discomfort or pain in the gastro-intestinal tract resulting from eating. It can result as much from emotional factors as from the passage of indigestible foods.

The process of absorption

IN THE MOUTH

No significant absorption occurs through the lining of the mouth.

IN THE STOMACH

The following simple substances can pass through the lining of the stomach into the blood stream in small quantities:
(a) water
(b) alcohol
(c) sugars
(d) minerals which are soluble in water, such as sodium chloride (salt)
(e) vitamins which are soluble in water, i.e. B-vitamins (but not vitamin B_{12}, which can only be absorbed in the ileum with the aid of the intrinsic factor produced by the stomach) and vitamin C.

IN THE SMALL INTESTINE

Almost all the absorption of nutrients occurs through the walls of the small intestine. Most of the water, alcohol, simple sugars, minerals and water-soluble vitamins are absorbed here too, as well as the digestion products of the energy-producing nutrients. These are:
(a) peptides and amino acids from proteins
(b) fatty acids from fats
(c) disaccharides from starch.
    Fat-soluble vitamins are absorbed in association with the fatty acids.
    Absorption into the cells of the intestinal wall is remarkably efficient; indeed, more than half of the small intestine can be removed without major consequences. The surface of the wall contains innumerable projections, called *villi*, which present a very large surface area (20–40 m² in total) for absorption. This process occurs both passively (by diffusion) and actively (when specific nutrients are drawn into cells already containing large amounts of those nutrients).
    Absorption can, however, be impaired. In coeliac disease the villi are lost. Substances such as laxatives and fibre which speed the passage of the

intestinal contents may reduce absorption in general. The fibre and phytic acid present in wholemeal cereals may also reduce the absorption of specific minerals including calcium, iron and zinc.

IN THE LARGE INTESTINE

The main functions of the large intestine are to absorb water from the residue moving through it from the small intestine, and to store the resultant faeces until they are expelled through the anus. Faeces are 70–80 per cent water, but also contain the undigested materials of food. The solid portion consists of fibre, debris from the continuously replaced cells of the intestinal wall including intestinal bacteria, and a small amount of undigested food. The entire passage of food from mouth to anus takes from 1 to 3 days, but it can be decreased by disease or by antibiotics which kill the intestinal bacteria, or it can be increased to as long as a week by diets very low in fibre.

The fate of major nutrients in the body

CARBOHYDRATES

The disaccharides entering the intestinal wall are split into monosaccharides which are carried by the bloodstream directly to the liver. They may then be:
(a) delivered as glucose to all the cells of the body to be used directly for energy via a series of controlled steps which produce carbon dioxide and water
(b) converted into glycogen and stored in the liver and skeletal muscles as a readily available source of energy
(c) converted into fatty acids and stored in the body fat (adipose tissue) as a source of energy.

The hormone *insulin* is required for the cellular metabolism of glucose, but fructose and dietary sorbitol (which is converted in the body into fructose) do not require insulin for their metabolism.

FATS

Almost all the fatty acids which enter the intestinal wall are immediately rebuilt into triglycerides which are carried to the bloodstream by lymph. Fat, in the form of microscopic particles called *chylomicrons*, circulates in the blood plasma which has a milky appearance for some time after a large meal is eaten. When fat reaches tissues requiring energy, fatty acids are released from it by enzymes and taken up into the cells. Fat may be further transformed by the liver, and most is finally deposited in the adipose tissue. Dietary fat is more easily converted into body fat than is the carbohydrate in food. The body's reservoir of fat is constantly available as a source of energy via another series of controlled steps which also give rise to carbon dioxide and water.

When the peptides enter the intestinal wall they are split into amino acids which are carried in the blood directly to the liver. They may then be:

(a) passed into the general circulation where they enter the body's 'pool' of indispensable and dispensable amino acids. These are then built into the structural proteins and specific enzymes which each cell needs.

(b) converted into those amino acids which are in short supply

(c) oxidized for energy, in some cases after conversion into glucose, if there is a residual excess of amino acids. Urea is also formed and excreted through the kidneys. If the diet as a whole is inadequate in energy, then a greater proportion of the protein will be used for this purpose in order to keep the body alive.

Control of nutrients in the blood

Blood is the means by which most nutrients are carried to and from the cells where they are needed. The concentration of most nutrients in the blood is normally controlled automatically as described in Chapters 7 and 8. In addition, when carbohydrate is eaten, the resulting slight increase in blood glucose is soon reduced by the hormone insulin. In *diabetes*, however, the pancreas does not secrete sufficient insulin, and the blood glucose concentration increases until the excess is excreted by the kidneys into the urine. In 'insulin-dependent' diabetes, this imbalance is so severe that insulin must be injected, but other forms of diabetes can usually be controlled by dietary regulation leading to a reduction in body weight.

7 Minerals

Most if not all of the inorganic elements or minerals can be detected in the body, but only about 15 of them are known to be essential and must be derived from food. Minute amounts of a further five or more are necessary for normal life in other animal species, and may well prove to be necessary for humans; it is difficult, however, to conceive of a dietary deficiency of these. Minerals have three main functions:

(a) as constituents of the bones and teeth. These include *calcium, phosphorus* and *magnesium.*

(b) as soluble salts which help to control the composition of body fluids and cells. These include *sodium* and *chloride* in the fluids outside the cells (e.g. blood), and *potassium*, magnesium and phosphorus inside the cells.

(c) as essential adjuncts to many enzymes, and other proteins such as haemoglobin, which are necessary for the release and utilisation of energy. *Iron*, phosphorus and *zinc*, and most of the other elements described at the end of this chapter, act in this way.

The eight elements mentioned above are in general needed in the greatest amounts in the diet or are present in the largest amounts in the body tissues (Table 9); these, together with sulphur which is mainly present as part of the amino acids methionine and cysteine, may be considered as the *major minerals*. The remainder, including chromium, cobalt, copper, fluoride, iodine, manganese, molybdenum and selenium, are equally important but are needed in smaller quantities. They are called *trace elements*. Most of these can be poisonous in excess.

Major minerals

IRON

Function, and effects of deficiency

The healthy adult body contains 3–4 g of iron, more than half of which is in the form of haemoglobin, the red pigment of blood. Iron is also present in the muscle protein myoglobin, and is stored to some extent in organs such as the liver. This store is an important source of iron for the first six months of an infant's life because the amount of iron in milk is small. Iron plays a major part in the body's use of oxygen: haemoglobin transports oxygen from the lungs to

Table 9. Daily intake and total body content of minerals for an adult man.

	Daily intake	Total body content
Major minerals		
Calcium	0.9 g	1 000 g
Phosphorus	1.5 g	780 g
Potassium	3.2 g	140 g
Sodium	3.4 g	140 g
Chloride	5.2 g	95 g
Magnesium	0.3 g	19 g
Iron	14.0 mg	4.2 g
Zinc	11.4 mg	2.3 g
Trace elements		
Fluoride	1.82[a] mg	2.6 g
Copper	1.63 mg	72 mg
Selenium	0.06 mg	>15 mg
Iodine	0.24 mg	13 mg
Manganese	5.0 mg	12 mg
Chromium	0.09 mg	Less than 2 mg
Cobalt	0.3 mg	1.5 mg

Intakes are likely to be far greater than requirements. A variable proportion is actually absorbed into the body (ranging from almost 100 per cent for sodium and chloride down to 5–10 per cent for iron, copper, manganese and probably chromium and cobalt too); the amount absorbed normally balances the amount lost in urine and sweat, except where increased retention is necessary during growth.

[a] Intakes of fluoride may be much higher in those people who drink large volumes of tea made with fluoridated water.

the tissues, and other iron-containing substances utilise the oxygen within the cells.

In Britain the average adult daily iron intake from all sources is 14 mg for men and 12 mg for women. These values are above the Reference Nutrient Intake (p. 69) for men, but below that for women, many of whom have increased iron needs due to menstrual blood losses. Adult women were reported in 1990 to obtain, on average, 15 per cent of their total intake from dietary supplements, but men obtained almost all their iron from food. If food provides insufficient iron to replace the body's losses, the stores are gradually depleted. Eventually anaemia results. Anaemia can also arise from a number of other causes including deficiencies of folic acid and vitamin B_{12}; cures are best effected medically and not nutritionally, for example by the use of iron salts which can be absorbed in much larger amounts than the iron from food.

Absorption and excretion

The amount of iron in the body is controlled almost entirely by the amount absorbed, because losses occur only when blood or other whole cells are lost in the general wear and tear of life. Losses do not occur at the end of the red blood corpuscle's life of 3–4 months, because the iron from them is efficiently re-utilised.

The extent to which iron from food is absorbed depends on whether it is in the form of haem or non-haem iron. The absorption of non-haem iron, but not haem iron, is influenced by the body's iron status and by the combination of foods ingested. Haem iron, which is the form occurring in the red pigments of meat and offals, is relatively well (20–30 per cent) absorbed. The non-haem iron occurring in cereals, pulses, vegetables, fruits, eggs and dairy products is generally less well absorbed, but absorption increases when the body's stores are depleted and when needs are greatest, as in growing children or menstruating or pregnant women. Its absorption also depends on other factors in the diet, e.g. it is increased by the presence of meat and by vitamin C, but decreased by the tannins in tea and by some forms of fibre.

Sources

About fifty per cent of the iron in the British diet comes from cereals and cereal products and about fourteen per cent from meat. The total amounts of iron present in selected foods are shown in Table 10.

Table 10. Total iron content of selected foods (edible portion).

	(mg/100 g)		(mg/100 g)
Milk, whole	0.1	Potatoes, old, boiled	0.4
Eggs, boiled	1.9	Watercress	2.2
Beef, stewing steak, stewed	3.0	Okra, boiled	0.6
Beefburgers, fried	3.1	Apricots, semi-dried, as eaten	3.4
Chicken, roast, meat only	0.8	Bread, white	1.6
Kidney, pig's, stewed	6.4	Bread, wholemeal	2.7
Liver, lamb's, fried	10.0	Cornflakes, fortified	6.7
Liver paté	7.1	Curry powder	58.3
Cod, fillet, baked	0.4	Soy sauce	2.7
Sardines, in tomato sauce	4.6	Cocoa powder	10.5
Courgettes, boiled	0.6	Chocolate, plain	2.4
Lettuce	0.7	Wine, red	0.9
Cabbage, boiled	0.3	Wine, white, dry	0.5

The main sources of iron in the diet are meat, breakfast cereals, bread and vegetables.

Function, and effects of deficiency

Calcium is the most abundant mineral in the body. All but about 1 per cent of it occurs in the bones and teeth, together with more than three-quarters of the body's phosphorus, in the form of calcium phosphates deposited in an organic framework. In addition to giving strength to the bones, these minerals act as a reserve supply for other needs and the calcium is constantly withdrawn into and replaced from the blood at carefully controlled rates. The remaining 5–10 g of calcium are essential for the contraction of muscles, including the heart muscle, for nerve function, for the activity of several enzymes, and for normal clotting of the blood.

The average intake of calcium in Britain from household food is more than 800 mg per day which is adequate for the needs of most people. Adult men and women consume on average 940 and 730 mg per day, respectively. Too little calcium in the bodies of young children results in stunted growth and in rickets (where the leg bones are deformed). In adults, the deficiency may show as osteomalacia (decalcified bones). The primary deficiency in rickets and osteomalacia, however, is of vitamin D so that too little calcium is absorbed. It occurs among some ethnic groups and in elderly people (especially those who are housebound) who remain indoors or wear enveloping clothes. Such people have a low exposure to sunlight and consequently form little or no vitamin D in their skin (p. 64). They may also be eating diets low in calcium or high in phytate (see below). Women who lose large quantities of calcium through repeated pregnancies and lactation are also at risk of osteomalacia.

As people age, their bone density decreases through losses of all components, not only calcium. This decline is particularly rapid in women about the time of the menopause. Large losses of bone lead to a condition, most common in elderly women, known as osteoporosis in which the bones are brittle and easily fractured. The basic cause of osteoporosis is unknown and studies are continuing into the role of nutrition in a disease that is costly in terms of suffering, disability and the need for health care of the elderly. However, it is wise for young people below the age of 30 to obtain plenty of dietary calcium and to take plenty of exercise to aid maximum bone development.

Absorption and excretion

Only 30–40 per cent of the calcium in the diet is normally absorbed and the remainder is lost in the faeces. But without adequate amounts of vitamin D, little or no calcium can be absorbed, and when fibre or phytic acid (present mainly in the outer layers of cereals) or oxalate (present in spinach and rhubarb) is added to the diet, calcium absorption is also reduced. It was partly to compensate for this that calcium carbonate was added to the high-extraction flour used during and after World War II; it is still added to all flour except wholemeal although it is now known that the body can adapt to the presence of phytic acid.

Excretion of absorbed calcium is mainly through the kidneys, and is increased when the diet contains large amounts of protein; some calcium is also lost in sweat. Adults normally absorb enough calcium to balance these losses until middle age unless they are immobilized, but pregnant and lactating women and growing children who are forming new bone must obtain more.

Sources

Few foods besides milk, yogurt and cheese and, in the UK, most bread (p. 133), contain significant amounts of calcium. It is therefore important that these foods are included in the diet, especially for children and adolescents. The extra calcium needed for lactation seems to be met from body stores, irrespective of dietary intake. However, many people consider it sensible to recommend extra calcium during lactation as a precaution. Reduced-fat milks contain essentially the same quantity of calcium as whole milk (see Table 11). However, children below the age of two need an energy-dense diet and should be given whole milk.

Table 11. Calcium content of selected foods (edible portion).

	(mg/100 g)		(mg/100 g)
Milk, whole	115	Courgettes, boiled	19
Milk, semi-skimmed	120	Cabbage, boiled	33
Milk, skimmed	120	Okra, boiled	120
Milk, dried, skimmed	1280	Onions, fried	47
Yogurt, low fat, fruit	150	Potatoes, old, boiled	5
Fromage frais, plain	89	Watercress	170
Cheese, Cheddar	720	Apples	4
Ice cream, non-dairy	120	Sultanas	64
Eggs, boiled	57	Peanuts, dry, roasted	52
Beef, stewing steak, stewed	15	Bread, white	110
Cod, fillet, baked	22	Bread, wholemeal	54
Sardines – canned in oil		Rice, white, boiled	18
(fish only)	550		
Baked beans	53		

The main sources of calcium in the diet are milk, cheese, bread and vegetables. For some people, hard water and the bones in canned sardines and salmon can be important.

Phosphorus is the second most abundant mineral in the body and, in the form of various phosphates, has a wide variety of essential functions. Calcium phosphates provide the strength of the bones and teeth, and inorganic phosphates are a major constituent of all cells. Phosphates play an essential role in the liberation and utilisation of energy from food. They are also constituents of nucleic acids and some fats, proteins and carbohydrates, and must be combined with some B-vitamins in the body before the latter can be active.

Because phosphorus is present in nearly all foods (Table 12), dietary deficiency is unknown in humans. Furthermore, phosphates are added to a number of processed foods. High intakes of phosphorus in the first few days of life, resulting from the use of unmodified cow's milk, may produce low levels of calcium in the blood, and muscular spasms (tetany). This milk has a high ratio of phosphorus to calcium compared with human milk, and the calcium present in it may combine with the fat present and be poorly absorbed.

Table 12. Phosphorus and magnesium content of selected foods (edible portion).

	Phosphorus (mg/100 g)	Magnesium (mg/100 g)
Milk, whole	92	11
Cheese, Cheddar	490	25
Eggs, whole, boiled	200	12
Beef, stewing steak, stewed	160	21
Chicken, roast, meat only	210	24
Ham, canned	280	18
Cod, fillets, baked	190	26
Sardines, in tomato sauce	400	51
Cabbage, boiled	25	4
Potatoes, old, boiled	31	14
Oranges	21	10
Peanuts, dry, roasted	420	190
Bread, white	91	24
Bread, wholemeal	200	76
Chapati, made without fat	120	37
Marmite	1700	180

The main sources of phosphorus in the diet are milk and milk products, bread and other cereal products, and meat and meat products. The main sources of magnesium are milk, bread and other cereal products, potatoes, and other vegetables.

Most of the magnesium in the body is present in the bones, but it is also an essential constituent of all cells and is necessary for the functioning of some of the enzymes which are involved in energy utilisation. Magnesium is widespread in foods (see Table 12), especially those of vegetable origin because it is an essential constituent of chlorophyll. Less than half is normally absorbed and, unlike the chemically related element calcium, this process is unaffected by vitamin D. In 1997, houshold food provided on average 226 mg magnesium per day. Deficiency is rare, and results from excessive losses in diarrhoea rather than from low intakes. No additional magnesium is required during pregnancy, but an extra 50 mg per day is needed during lactation to offset secretion in breast milk.

ZINC

Zinc helps with the healing of wounds, and is also associated with the activity of a wide variety of enzymes; about one-third of the comparatively large amount which is present in the body is in the bones. Zinc is present in a wide range of foods, particularly in association with protein, and meat and dairy products are excellent sources. About one-third of the zinc in the diet as a whole is absorbed, but this is reduced if large amounts of whole cereals rich in dietary fibre and phytic acid are eaten, although the amount of zinc present in wholegrain cereals is enough to offset this. Average adult intakes are between 9 and 12 mg per day. High intakes from water stored in galvanised containers have caused toxicity. The zinc content of selected foods is shown in Table 13.

Table 13. Zinc content of selected foods (edible portion).

	Zinc (mg/100 g)
Milk	0.4
Cheese, Cheddar	2.3
Beef, stewing steak, stewed	8.7
Chicken, roast, meat only	1.5
Ham, canned	2.3
Paté, liver	2.9
Cod, fillets, baked	0.5
Eggs, whole, boiled	1.3
Potatoes, old, boiled	0.3
Bread, white	0.6
Bread, wholemeal	1.8
Chapati, made without fat	1.0

The main sources of zinc in the diet are meat and meat products, milk, bread, and other cereal products.

Functions, and effects of deficiency and excess

All body fluids contain salt (sodium chloride), but especially those fluids outside the cells such as blood. These elements are involved in maintaining the water balance of the body, and sodium is also essential for muscle and nerve activity.

Salt requirements are closely related to water requirements, and too low an intake results in muscular cramps. Salt intake may, however, have to be severely restricted in certain kidney diseases or where there is marked water retention. Very young infants also cannot tolerate high sodium intakes because their kidneys cannot excrete the excess, so salt should not be added to infants' diets. Habitually high sodium intakes can be associated with high blood pressure.

Absorption and excretion

It is essential for life that the concentration of sodium and chloride in the blood is maintained within close limits. As an excess of (added) salt in the diet is readily absorbed, control of sodium in the blood is achieved by its excretion through the kidneys into the urine. There is also a variable loss through sweat. This is only significant after strenuous exercise or in hot climates, as for miners in deep pits, steel workers and athletes, and although adaptation can occur, extra salt may still be needed to prevent muscle cramps.

The average sodium intake from all sources by adults of 3.5 g per day (equivalent to about 9 g per day of salt) is well above what is needed to maintain normal functions in a temperate climate. In order to help lower the average blood pressure of the population, and so decrease the prevalence of coronary heart disease and stroke, current recommendations are for the average sodium intake of adults to decrease by about one-third, that is to about 2.3 g sodium (6 g salt) per day.

Sources

Sodium and chloride are comparatively low in all foods which have not been processed, but salt is added to very many prepared foods. For example, salt is low in pork and other meats, but high in bacon, sausages and most other meat products; low in herrings, but high in kippers. Salt is also added to canned vegetables, most butter, margarine, cheese, bread, many savoury snack foods and some breakfast cereals during manufacture, and to many foods during home cooking and on the plate. Sodium may also be derived from sodium bicarbonate and monosodium glutamate. Table 14 shows the amounts of sodium in selected foods.

Table 14. Sodium and potassium content of selected foods as bought (edible portion).

	Sodium (mg/100 g)	Potassium (mg/100 g)
Milk, semi-skimmed	55	150
Cheese, Cheddar	670	77
Eggs, whole, raw	140	130
Beef, mince, raw	86	290
Corned beef, canned	950	140
Bacon, streaky	1500	240
Chicken	81	320
Sausages, pork	760	160
Haddock, fresh	120	300
Haddock, smoked	1220	290
Butter, unsalted	11	15
Butter, salted	750	15
Margarine	800	5
Low-fat spread	650	110
Potatoes, old	7	360
Potato crisps	1070	1060
Peas, frozen	3	190
Peas, canned, processed	380	150
Tomatoes, raw	9	250
Orange juice	2	180
Bananas	1	400
Peaches, canned in juice	12	170
Raisins	60	1020
Bread, white	520	110
Bread, wholemeal	550	230
Cornflakes	1110	100
Muesli, Swiss style	380	440
Coffee, instant, granules	41	4000
Marmite	4500	2600
Soy sauce	5720	360
Gravy instant granules	6330	150

The sodium content of vegetables is much higher if they are cooked in salted water. Apart from this, the main sources of sodium in the UK diet are table salt, bread and cereal products, meat products including bacon and ham, and milk. The main sources of potassium are vegetables, meat and milk. Fruit and fruit juices are also noteworthy as being much richer in potassium than sodium.

POTASSIUM

Function, and effects of deficiency

Potassium is present largely in the fluids within the body cells where its concentration is carefully controlled. The total amount in the body is closely related to the amount of lean tissue. Potassium has a complementary action with sodium in the functioning of cells.

As potassium is found so widely in foods, deficiency is unlikely to occur. Like sodium, most of the potassium in the diet is absorbed and the excess is excreted through the kidneys. Losses may be large if diuretics or purgatives are frequently taken, and in cases of protein-energy malnutrition (*kwashiorkor*) where tissue breakdown as well as diarrhoea occurs. Potassium is essential to the correct functioning of heart muscle and in severe cases of potassium depletion, heart failure may result unless supplements are given.

Higher intakes of potassium may counter the effects of sodium and help to lower blood pressure and decrease the risk of stroke. It is currently recommended, therefore, that the average adult intake of potassium should increase from 3 g to 3.5 g per day.

Sources

Potassium is widespread in foods, but is particularly abundant in potatoes, vegetables, fruit (especially bananas) and juices (Table 14).

Trace elements

Knowledge of the exact roles and dietary requirements for some of the following minerals is incomplete for three reasons: they have only recently been found to be essential; dietary deficiencies of many are unknown; and the utilisation of one may be affected by the amounts of other elements present.

COBALT

Cobalt can be utilised by humans only as part of vitamin B_{12} (p. 58). Average intakes are 0.3 mg per day. Very high doses (29.5 mg per day), which were used in the treatment of certain anaemias, have proved toxic.

COPPER

Copper is associated with a number of enzymes. Deficiency has occasionally been observed in malnourished infants, particularly if their initial stores were depleted by prolonged feeding of cow's milk alone (which contains less copper than most foods). Although shellfish and liver are particularly rich in copper, the main sources in the average diet are meat, bread and other cereal products, and vegetables. Intakes of copper by British adults are on average about 1.4 mg per day.

CHROMIUM

Chromium is involved in the utilisation of glucose. It is fairly widely distributed in foods; those with a high content include brewer's yeast, meat, wholegrain cereals, legumes and nuts. A safe level of intake is believed to be more than 25 µg per day for adults and between 0.1 and 1.0 µg per kg per day for children and adolescents.

FLUORIDE

Fluoride is associated with the structure of bones and teeth, and increases the resistance of the latter to decay. Drinking water is an important source, but the natural content is variable and is often below the optimum level of 1 mg per litre (1 part per million). The only other important sources of fluoride in the diet are tea and seafood (especially fish whose bones are eaten). The use of a fluoridated toothpaste helps to prevent dental caries.

IODINE

Iodine is an essential constituent of hormones produced by the thyroid gland in the neck, and most of the iodine in the body is in this gland. Deficiency causes it to enlarge – a condition known as *goitre*. The richest source of iodine is seafood. The amount of iodine in vegetable and cereal foods depends on the level in the soil, and that in foods from animal sources depends on the level in their diet. Because of the widespread use of iodine in animal feed, milk and dairy products are now the main sources of iodine in the British diet, and meat and eggs are also important. The use of iodised table salt, although not common in the UK, is beneficial in areas where goitre is prevalent, whether it results from low intakes of iodine itself or from reduced absorption caused by goitrogens in vegetables from the cabbage family. The average adult intake in the UK is about 200 µg per day. Low average intakes of about 80 µg per day have been found in vegans. Edible seaweeds, which are rich in iodine, could be a useful source for vegans if used in moderation. Excessive intakes of iodine can have toxic effects on the thyroid.

MANGANESE

Manganese is present in a number of enzymes and activates others. Tea is exceptionally rich in manganese, and plant products, including nuts, spices and whole cereals are in general much better sources of manganese than animal products.

MOLYBDENUM

Molybdenum is essential for the functioning of enzymes involved in DNA metabolism. Possible deficiency has only been reported in adults fed much lower levels than in UK diets.

Selenium is needed for an enzyme in the red blood cells, and the main dietary sources are meat, fish and cereal products. The selenium content of plants varies widely with the level in the soil, and in some parts of the world animals fed on local produce develop symptoms of deficiency or excess. Selenium intakes in the UK population as a whole are falling. This is thought to be due in part to the trend over the last 25 years towards using European wheat, which has a low selenium content, rather than North American wheat for bread making. Additionally, the overall consumption of cereal foods, most notably bread, has declined in the last 20 years. Current estimated intakes of selenium are 29–39µg per day which are below the LRNI (see page 68 and Table 25). COMA concluded in 1997 that there is no evidence at present of adverse health consequences from current intakes. COMA will consider the issue further when more data is available.

8 Vitamins

Until the beginning of the 20th century, it was believed that the only components of a diet necessary for health, growth and reproduction were pure proteins, fats, carbohydrates and a number of inorganic elements. This view had to be changed when it was found that minute amounts of additional materials were also essential. These could be extracted from a variety of foods and appeared to be of two types: fat-soluble ('A') and water-soluble ('B'). They were later each discovered to contain several active components, or vitamins. The former are mainly associated with fatty foods and include vitamins A, D, E and K. The latter embraces the vitamins of the B complex and includes thiamin (B_1), riboflavin (B_2), niacin (or nicotinic acid), folate, vitamin B_6, vitamin B_{12}, biotin and pantothenic acid. Vitamin C is also water-soluble, but often occurs in different foods from the B-vitamins. Many of these vitamins exist in more than one chemical form.

The absence of a vitamin from the diet or, more usually, its presence in insufficient amounts, leads to both general and specific symptoms. The most common general symptoms are, as with deficiencies of many other components of the diet, a feeling of malaise and restriction of the growth of children. The specific symptoms of deficiency in humans are discussed separately for each vitamin. Excessive intakes of most water-soluble vitamins either from vitamin pills or from very unusual diets have little effect as they are rapidly excreted in the urine. However, very high intakes of some, such as vitamin B_6 and niacin, can have adverse effects. Excessive intakes of fat-soluble vitamins accumulate in the body and can also be dangerous. For example, high levels of vitamin A may have undesirable effects on the unborn child if consumed during pregnancy (see below).

Factors affecting the stability of vitamins in foods are discussed elsewhere (see pp. 82–3).

Vitamin A

The chemical name of vitamin A is *retinol*. Retinol itself is found only in foods of animal origin, but milk and many fruits and vegetables also contain the deep yellow or orange *carotenes* which can be converted in the body to retinol and are therefore sources of vitamin A activity. The most important of these is beta-carotene. The most convenient way of expressing the total vitamin A activity of a diet is as *retinol equivalents*: by convention, 1 µg retinol equivalent is equal to 1 µg retinol or 6 µg beta-carotene.[1] This average value takes into account the conversion losses and the lesser absorption of beta-carotene compared with retinol in the general diet.

Function, and effects of deficiency or excess

Deficiency Vitamin A is essential for vision in dim light; thus prolonged deficiency (sufficient to deplete any stores in the liver, which in previously well-nourished people will last for 1 to 2 years) results in night blindness. In children in many parts of the world deficiency also results in severe eye lesions (xerophthalmia) and complete blindness (keratomalacia). Vitamin A is also necessary for the maintenance of healthy skin and surface tissues, especially those which excrete mucus.

Excess Excessive doses, for example from taking large amounts of vitamin A preparations for long periods, accumulate in the liver and can be poisonous. There is also an association between very high levels of retinol consumption during pregnancy and the incidence of some birth defects. As a matter of precaution therefore, women in the UK who are or might become pregnant are advised not to take vitamin A supplements except on the advice of their doctor and, as an additional precaution, not to eat liver or liver products since these can also be very rich sources of retinol.

Sources

Vitamin A is not widely distributed in food. Animals store vitamin A in their livers which are often extremely concentrated, but very variable, sources of retinol. Fish liver oils are also a very rich natural source of vitamin A. Kidneys, dairy produce and eggs contain substantial amounts, but lard and dripping contain none. Variable amounts of beta-carotene are found in carrots and dark green or yellow vegetables, roughly in proportion to the depth of their colour; thus dark plants such as spinach contain more than cabbage, and the dark outer leaves of a cabbage contain more than the pale inner heart. Furthermore, all margarine for retail sale is required by law to contain about the same amount of vitamin A as butter (see p. 100). This is now added to margarines and reduced-fat spreads (although not by law for the latter) in the form of synthetic retinol and beta-carotene.

---

[1] The amounts of vitamin A in foods are sometimes quoted in international units (IU). To convert these to µg retinol equivalents, multiply the IU of retinol (in foods of animal origin) by 0.3, and divide the IU of beta-carotene (in foods of plant origin) by 10. (This is because 1 IU vitamin A = 0.3 µg retinol or 0.6 µg beta-carotene; and 1 µg retinol equivalent = 1 µg retinol or 6 µg beta-carotene).

The amounts of vitamin A in selected foods are shown in Table 15. The British diet as a whole provides well above the Reference Nutrient Intake (see p. 69) of this vitamin. On average about two thirds come from retinol itself, with 22 per cent of this from liver alone, and the remaining third from carotene.

Table 15. Vitamin A content of selected foods (edible portion).

Animal foods	Retinol (µg/100 g)
Milk, whole	55[a]
Milk, semi-skimmed	23[a]
Milk, skimmed	1
Cheese, Cheddar	363
Eggs, whole, boiled	190
Beef, stewing steak, stewed	0
Liver, lamb's, fried	22960[a]
Kidney, pig's, stewed	46
Cod, fillets, baked	2
Mackerel, smoked	25
Sardines, canned, fish only	11
Butter	887[a]
Margarine	905[b]
Cod liver oil	18000

Vegetable foods	Beta-carotene[c] (µg/100 g)	Retinol equivalents (µg/100 g)
Potatoes, old, boiled	0	0
Sweetpotato, yellow flesh, boiled	3960	660
Cabbage, boiled	210	35
Spinach, boiled	3840	640
Peas, fresh, boiled	250	42
Peas, frozen, boiled	405	67
Carrots, old, boiled	7560	1260
Tomatoes, raw	640	105
Peppers, capsicum, red, raw	3840	640
Peppers, capsicum, green, raw	265	45
Apricots, semi-dried, as eaten	545	91
Mango	1800	300
Bread	0	0

[a] Includes some retinol equivalents.
[b] Some types, which do not contain beta-carotene have lower levels than this.
[c] Beta-carotene content of many vegetables and fruit varies widely depending on variety and season.
The main sources of vitamin A in the diet are liver, carrots, margarine, butter and low-fat spreads and milk.

B-vitamins

Although the chemical structure of each of the B-vitamins is quite different, they have several features in common. They act as 'co-factors' in different enzyme systems in the body. They tend to occur in the same foods and, being water-soluble, they are not stored for long in the body. These characteristics mean that diets containing too little of the B-vitamins can lead to *multiple* deficiency diseases within a few months.

THIAMIN (VITAMIN B₁)

Function, and effects of deficiency

Thiamin is necessary for the steady and continuous release of energy from carbohydrate. Thiamin requirements are thus related to the amount of carbohydrate, and more or less to the amount of energy, in the diet. The deficiency disease, beriberi, results from a diet which is not only poor in thiamin but also rich in carbohydrate (or alcohol), such as one based almost entirely on polished rice from which the thiamin-rich seedcoat has been removed.

Sources

Thiamin is widely distributed in both animal and vegetable foods (Table 16). Good sources are those which contain more than 0.1 mg per 1000 kJ (0.04 mg per 100 kcal), such as milk, offal, pork, eggs, vegetables and fruit, wholegrain cereals and fortified breakfast cereals. It should, however, be noted that cooking may result in considerable losses from these foods (p. 82). Fats, sugars and alcoholic drinks contain no thiamin at all.

Wheat in the form of bread has long been a major source of carbohydrate in the British diet, but much of the thiamin is removed with the bran in the milling necessary to produce white bread. Thus one 30 g (about 1 oz) slice of wholemeal bread provides 0.10 mg thiamin (0.37 mg per 1000 kJ; 0.16 mg per 100 kcal), while 30 g of unfortified white bread would provide only about 0.03 mg thiamin (0.1 mg per 1000 kJ; 0.04 mg per 100 kcal). It is therefore a legal requirement in the UK that all flour except wholemeal be fortified with thiamin to at least 0.24 mg per 100 g, equivalent to about 0.17 mg per 1000 kJ (0.07 mg per 100 kcal; see pp. 93–4).

RIBOFLAVIN (VITAMIN B₂)

Function, and effects of deficiency

Riboflavin is a bright yellow substance, which is essential for the utilisation of energy from food. Specific deficiency signs are rarely seen in humans, but include sores in the corners of the mouth.

Table 16. Thiamin content of selected foods.

	Thiamin (mg/100 g)	Thiamin (mg/1000 kJ)
Milk, whole	0.03	0.11
Bacon, streaky, fried	0.37	0.18
Beef, stewing steak, stewed	0.03	0.03
Corned beef, canned	0.00	0.00
Chicken, roast, meat only	0.08	0.13
Pork chop, grilled	0.66	0.48
Sausage, pork, fried	0.01	0.01
Sugar	0.00	0.00
Peas, frozen, boiled	0.26	0.89
Potatoes, old, boiled	0.18	0.59
Lentils, boiled	0.11	0.26
Oranges	0.11	0.70
Pineapple, canned in juice	0.09	0.45
Peanuts, dry roasted	0.18	0.07
Bread, white, average	0.21	0.21
Bread, wholemeal, average	0.34	0.37
Chapati, made without fat	0.23	0.27
Cornflakes, fortified	1.00	0.65
Rice, easy cook, white, boiled	0.01	0.02
Rice, brown, boiled	0.14	0.23
Spaghetti, white, boiled	0.01	0.02
Spaghetti, wholemeal, boiled	0.21	0.43
Marmite	3.10	4.25
Lager	0.00	0.00

The main sources of thiamin in the diet are bread and cereal products, potatoes, milk and meat.

Sources

Although riboflavin is widely distributed in foods, especially those of animal origin (Table 17), about 40 per cent of the average intake in Britain is derived from one source alone – milk and its products. Some people in the UK, such as vegans, who avoid milk, have low intakes. As riboflavin is destroyed by sunlight, bottled milk should not be allowed to stay too long on the doorstep.

NIACIN

Function, and effects of deficiency or excess

Nicotinic acid and nicotinamide are two forms of another B-vitamin (known collectively as niacin) which is involved in the utilisation of food energy. Deficiency results in pellagra, in which the skin becomes dark and scaly especially where it is exposed to light. Pharmacological doses of nicotinic acid (but not nicotinamide) can cause burning sensations in the face and hands, and have been associated with liver damage in some people.

Table 17. Riboflavin content of selected foods (edible portion).

	Riboflavin (mg/100 g)
Milk	0.17
Cheese, Cheddar	0.40
Beef, stewing steak, stewed	0.33
Chicken, roast, meat only	0.19
Liver, lamb's, fried	4.40
Kidney, pig's, stewed	2.10
Eggs, whole, boiled	0.35
Potatoes, old, boiled	0.01
Brussels sprouts, boiled	0.09
Mushrooms, fried	0.34
Banana	0.06
Rice, white, boiled	0.00
Bread, white	0.06
Cornflakes, fortified	1.30
Tea, infusion	0.01
Marmite	11.00

The main sources of riboflavin in the diet are milk, meat, fortified cereal products, and egg.

Sources

There are two apparent anomalies associated with pellagra: it occurs when the diet consists largely of maize, a cereal which contains nicotinic acid; and it can be cured by milk or eggs which are not rich sources of this vitamin. The reasons for these anomalies are firstly, that the nicotinic acid in maize and other cereals is largely present in a bound form which is unavailable to humans (although it can be released by alkali as in the preparation of Mexican tortillas), and secondly, that proteins of milk and eggs are especially rich in tryptophan – an amino acid which can be converted to nicotinic acid in the body.

It is therefore convenient to express the niacin content of foods in terms of equivalents: on average, 1 mg of niacin equivalent equals 1 mg of available niacin or 60 mg of tryptophan, and this is accepted as a definition. The amounts of both forms in selected foods are shown in Table 18.

PYRIDOXINE (VITAMIN B_6)

Function, and effects of deficiency or excess

Vitamin B_6, or pyridoxine, is involved in the metabolism of amino acids, including the conversion of tryptophan to niacin; the requirements are thus related to the protein content of the diet. The vitamin is also necessary for the

Table 18. Niacin equivalents in selected foods (edible portion).

	Total niacin (mg/100 g)	Tryptophan (mg/100 g)	Niacin equivalent[a] (mg/100 g)
Milk	0.1	42	0.8
Cheese, Cheddar	0.1	360	6.1
Beef, stewing steak, stewed	3.6	396	10.2
Pork chop, grilled	5.7	318	11.0
Chicken, roast, meat only	8.2	276	12.8
Cod, fillet, baked	1.7	240	5.7
Eggs, whole, boiled	0.1	222	3.8
Baked beans	0.5	48	1.3
Peas, frozen, boiled	1.6	54	2.5
Potatoes, old, boiled	0.5	24	0.9
Bread, white	1.7	102	3.4[b]
Bread, wholemeal	4.1	108	5.9[b]
Wheatgerm	4.5	318	9.8[b]
Tea, infusion	0.1	0	0.1
Coffee, instant, infusion	0.7	0	0.7

[a] Available niacin and (tryptophan ÷ 60)

[b] Naturally occurring nicotinic acid in cereals is considered unavailable, but white flour is fortified to at least 1.6 mg per 100 g by law. The main sources of niacin in the diet are meat and meat products, potatoes, bread and fortified breakfast cereals.

formation of haemoglobin. Deficiency is rare in humans and there is no evidence that women who are pregnant or taking oral contraceptives have requirements greater than other adults. Very high intakes (more than 50 mg per day), however, are potentially harmful as they can affect sensory nerve function. The Government's advice is that people should limit their intake from dietary supplements (i.e. vitamin and mineral pills) to no more than 10 mg per day unless acting on professional advice.

Sources

Vitamin B_6 occurs widely in food, especially in meat and fish, eggs, whole cereals and some vegetables (Table 19). Microorganisms in the intestine synthesise the vitamin, some of which may be available to the body.

VITAMIN B_{12}

Function, and effects of deficiency

Vitamin B_{12} is a mixture of several related compounds, all of which contain the trace element cobalt. Together with folate, it is needed by rapidly dividing cells such as those in the bone marrow which form blood cells. Deficiency leads to a characteristic (pernicious) anaemia and the degeneration of nerve cells. Because vitamin B_{12} does not occur in vegetable foods, deficiency may occur in vegans who do not consume meat, milk, eggs, nor any special

Table 19. Vitamin B$_6$ content of selected foods (edible portion).

	Vitamin B$_6$ (mg/100 g)
Milk	0.06
Beef, stewing steak, stewed	0.30
Chicken, roast, meat only	0.26
Turkey, roast, meat only	0.32
Cod, fillets, baked	0.38
Baked beans	0.14
Brussels sprouts, boiled	0.19
Peas, frozen, boiled	0.09
Potatoes, old, boiled	0.33
Yam, boiled	0.12
Oranges	0.10
Banana	0.29
Bread, white	0.07
Bread, wholemeal	0.12
Rice, white, boiled	0.07
Wheatgerm	3.30

The main sources of vitamin B$_6$ in the diet are potatoes and other vegetables, milk and meat.

supplement. It more usually arises, however, in those few individuals whose gastric juice contains no 'intrinsic factor' (p. 35) and who therefore cannot absorb this vitamin.

Sources

Vitamin B$_{12}$ occurs only in animal products and in microorganisms including yeast. Liver is the richest source, but useful amounts also occur in eggs, cheese, milk, meat and fish, and in fortified breakfast cereals, as shown in Table 20.

FOLATE

Function, and effects of deficiency

Folate (folic acid and various derivatives) has several functions, including its action with vitamin B$_{12}$ in rapidly dividing cells. Deficiency leads to a characteristic (megaloblastic) form of anaemia which must be distinguished from that caused by a deficiency of vitamin B$_{12}$. Folate deficiency can result not only from a poor diet, but also from increased needs for the synthesis of red blood cells in pregnant women, from increased requirements arising from certain medical conditions in the elderly and when there is decreased absorption of folate in gastro-intestinal disease.

59

Table 20. Vitamin B$_{12}$ content of selected foods (edible portion).

	Vitamin B$_{12}$ (µg/100 g)
Milk	0.4
Cheese, Cheddar	1.1
Eggs, whole, raw	2.5
Beef, lamb, pork, lean only, cooked	2.0
Liver, lamb's, fried	81.0
Paté, liver	7.2
Cod, fillets, baked	2.0
Cornflakes, fortified	1.7
Marmite	0.5

The main sources of vitamin B$_{12}$ in the diet are offals, other meat and meat products, and milk.

Women who increase their folic acid/folate intake before pregnancy and during its early stages can help to reduce their risk of having a baby with a neural tube defect (NTD) such as anencephaly or spina bifida, in which the brain or spinal cord or their protective coverings fail to develop properly. To reduce the risk of an occurrence of NTD, all women planning a pregnancy are advised to take a daily dietary supplement of 0.4 mg folic acid and eat plenty of folate-rich foods prior to conception and during the early months of pregnancy. To reduce the risk of recurrence of NTD, those who have already had an affected child should take a supplement of 4 or 5 mg folic acid daily before becoming pregnant and up to the twelfth week of pregnancy.

Sources

Folate occurs in small amounts in many foods. Rich sources are generally also rich in other B-vitamins. They include offal, yeast extract, green leafy vegetables and fortified foods such as some bread and many breakfast cereals. Most fruits, meat and dairy produce contain comparatively little. Folate is readily destroyed in cooking, much being lost in the water used for cooking vegetables, and it is also readily oxidised to unavailable forms of the vitamin. Thus care should be taken to include several good sources of folate in the diet and to cook vegetables in only a little water for a short time to minimise the risk of deficiency. Selected sources of folate are shown in Table 21.

PANTOTHENIC ACID

Pantothenic acid is necessary for the release of energy from fat and carbohydrate. Dietary deficiencies of this vitamin are unlikely in humans because it is

Table 21. Folate content of selected foods (edible portion).

	Folate (µg/100 g)
Fortified breakfast cereals	250
Bread, brown	40
Bread, white	29
Potatoes, boiled	26
Peas, frozen, boiled	47
Broccoli, boiled	64
Brussels sprouts, boiled	110
Lettuce	55
Okra, boiled	46
Apples, eating	1
Bananas	14
Oranges	31
Almonds	48
Peanuts	110
Blackeye beans, boiled	210
Chickpeas, boiled	54
Egg, chicken, boiled	39
Kidney, ox, stewed	75
Liver, ox, stewed	290
Beef, stewed	16
Cheese, Cheddar	33
Milk, semi-skimmed	6

The main sources of folate in the diet are potatoes, fortified breakfast cereals, bread and fresh vegetables.

so widespread in food. Animal products, cereals and legumes are especially rich sources.

BIOTIN

Biotin is essential for the metabolism of fat. Very small amounts are required, and sufficient may well be made by the bacteria normally inhabiting the large intestine. It is therefore probable that no additional biotin need be provided in the diet, except in the very unusual situation when large quantities of raw eggs are consumed. Raw, but not cooked, egg white contains a substance (avidin) which combines with biotin making it unavailable to the body.

Rich sources of biotin include offal and egg yolk. Smaller amounts are obtained from milk and dairy products, cereals, fish, fruit and vegetables.

Vitamin C (ascorbic acid)

Function, and effects of deficiency

Vitamin C is necessary for the maintenance of healthy connective tissue. Humans are among the few animals (along with monkeys and guinea pigs) unable to form their own vitamin C, and must therefore obtain it from food. Deficiency soon results in bleeding, especially from small blood vessels (capillaries) under the skin and from the gums, and wounds heal more slowly. Scurvy follows, and, if the deficiency is prolonged, death results. Mild deficiencies may occur in infants who are given unsupplemented cow's milk, in people eating poor diets (for example some elderly people), and in food faddists eating little but whole-grain cereals which lack vitamin C.

Claims that extremely large amounts of vitamin C (10–100 times the Reference Nutrient Intake) cure colds and other minor ailments have little scientific basis. Excessively high intakes can lead to diarrhoea in some people.

Sources

Vitamin C is not widely distributed in foods. Small amounts occur in milk, especially breast milk, and liver, but virtually all the vitamin C in most diets is derived from vegetables and fruit. Many people do not eat enough vegetables and fruit and vitamin C is readily lost from these foods during storage, preparation and cooking (p. 82). Care should be taken to include good sources of the vitamin in the diet to minimise the risk of deficiency. The average vitamin C content of selected foods is shown in Table 22.

Citrus fruits and blackcurrants are particularly rich sources, but some tropical fruits, such as guavas and West Indian cherries, are even richer. Synthetic vitamin C, which is equally valuable, may be added to fruit juices to compensate for losses during storage and to juice drinks which are only partially composed of fruit juice.

The amount of vitamin C in any particular fruit or vegetable may differ considerably from the value shown in the table. This is because of the natural variations which occur, the variable losses during the time between harvesting and consumption in the home, and the variations in cooking methods that may be used. As an example, fresh peas may contain between 10 and 30 mg per 100 g; the higher values would tend to occur in the spring and early summer when the plants are growing most rapidly, and may be preserved by freezing. The loss which can occur after harvesting is illustrated in Table 22 by the average change in vitamin C content of potatoes during storage; it can also be substantial in the days which elapse between the harvest of leafy vegetables and their consumption in the home. Vitamin C, like riboflavin, is also rapidly lost when milk is allowed to stand on the doorstep; this may be important for young children and those older people with restricted diets for whom milk may be one of the few sources of this vitamin.

Table 22. Vitamin C content of selected foods (edible portion).

	Raw (mg/100 g)	After boiling (mg/100 g)
Courgettes	21	11
Carrots	6	2
Cabbage, average	49	20
Cauliflower	43	27
Lettuce	5	
Pepper, green	120	
Plantain (green banana)	15	9
Potatoes, new, average	16	9
Potatoes, old, freshly dug	21	
stored 3 months	9	
stored 9 months	7	
average	11	6
Sweetpotatoes	23	17
Tomatoes, raw	17	
Apples	6	
Bananas	11	
Blackcurrants	200	115 (stewed)
Grapefruit juice	31	
Kiwi fruit	59	
Mango	37	
Oranges	54	

The main sources of vitamin C in the diet are fruit and fruit juices, potatoes and other vegetables. The vitamin C content of many vegetables and fruit varies widely, depending on variety, season and freshness.

The highest contributions to vitamin C intake in the UK are made by fresh fruit and fruit juices, but potatoes also contribute a significant amount as the large quantities eaten more than compensate for their comparatively modest content of this vitamin. Instant potato can contain as much as fresh potato if it has been fortified. The only vegetable materials containing no vitamin C are cereal grains (unless they are allowed to sprout) and dried peas and beans.

Vitamin D

Function, and effects of deficiency and excess

Vitamin D helps to maintain bone mineralisation by ensuring a plentiful supply of calcium in the blood. It achieves this primarily by enhancing the absorption of dietary calcium from the intestine, but it may also have a direct positive effect on the deposition of calcium in bone. Infants and children who are deprived of vitamin D develop rickets, with deformed bones which are too

63

weak to support their weight. Because these changes readily become permanent, it is important to prevent their development; hence in the UK and some other countries, preparations containing vitamin D are available for children and pregnant women, and margarine and many reduced-fat spreads and milk products are fortified. Some adolescents and women who are repeatedly pregnant and who breastfeed all their babies, and some elderly people, may also suffer from bone softening (osteomalacia) because they absorb too little calcium from a diet which is low in both calcium and vitamin D.

Too high an intake of vitamin D causes more calcium to be absorbed than can be excreted; the excess is then deposited in, and can damage, the kidneys. It is therefore necessary for vitamin D intakes to be carefully controlled, especially in young children.

Sources

Vitamin D is obtained both from the action of sunlight on a substance in the skin, and from the diet. Sunlight is by far the most important source for most people, who will need little or no extra from food. But several groups of people should ensure that their food contains sufficient vitamin D: children and pregnant and lactating women, whose requirements are especially high, and those who receive little exposure to sunlight such as older housebound people or members of certain ethnic communities who prefer to wear enveloping clothes.

Few foods contain vitamin D. All those which do so naturally are products of animal origin, and contain vitamin D_3 (cholecalciferol) derived as in humans from the action of sunlight on the animal's skin or from its own food. There may thus be seasonal variations in the amounts present. Vitamin D_3 is also used to fortify a number of foods, as (sometimes) is vitamin D_2 (ergocalciferol), which appears to be equally effective in humans and can readily be manufactured using plant materials. Vitamin D is required by law to be added to margarine for retail sale (p. 100) and is also added to most reduced-fat spreads. It is also included in the supplements provided (free to those in need) in the UK to pregnant and lactating women and to children up to 5 years old. Table 23 shows some food sources of vitamin D.

Vitamin E

Function, and effects of deficiency and excess

A number of related compounds (*tocopherols*) show vitamin E activity, the most potent being alpha-tocopherol. Its major activity in the body is as an antioxidant. Vitamin E occurs widely in foods including those eaten by the poorest of the world's peoples, and like other fat-soluble vitamins is stored in the body. For this reason deficiency is never seen except in two groups of people. Premature infants who have very low fat stores develop an anaemia

Table 23. Vitamin D content of selected foods (edible portion).

	Vitamin D (µg/100 g)
Milk, whole	0.03
Milk, skimmed	0.00
Milk, skimmed, dried, fortified	2.1
Evaporated milk	3.9
Cheese, Cheddar	0.3
Yogurt, low-fat, fruit	Tr
Eggs, whole, boiled	1.7
Beef, average, stewing steak	Tr
Liver, lamb's, fried	0.5
Herring and kipper, baked	25.0
Salmon, canned	12.5
Sardines, canned, drained	7.5
Butter	0.8
Margarine	7.9
Low-fat spread	8.0
Vegetable oil	0.0
Cornflakes, fortified	2.1
Malted milk drinks made with whole milk	0.3
Cod liver oil	210.0

The main sources of vitamin D in the diet are margarine, fatty fish, dairy and low-fat spreads, breakfast cereals and eggs.

when fed on formulas low in vitamin E and rich in the polyunsaturated fatty acids which increase the need for this vitamin. Manufacturers now ensure, therefore, that infant formulas contain sufficient vitamin E. People who cannot absorb or utilise the vitamin can also be deficient. Very high intakes do not appear to be toxic.

Sources

Most foods contain vitamin E. The richest sources are vegetable oil, nuts and seeds, some cereal products and egg yolk; animal fats and meat, fruit and vegetables contain comparatively little.

Vitamin K

Vitamin K is necessary for the normal clotting of blood. Deficiency is seen in a very few newborn babies so that all babies should be given a supplement of vitamin K at birth. It also occurs in rare individuals who cannot absorb or utilise the vitamin. A dietary deficiency is unlikely, partly because the vitamin is widespread in vegetable foods such as spinach, cabbage and cauliflower, peas and cereals, and partly because our intestinal bacteria can synthesise it.

Vitamins and antioxidant activity

Some carotenes (p. 52), vitamin C (p. 62) and vitamin E (p. 64) are among the many substances in food which can have antioxidant properties. This attribute can help to counter the effects of reactive oxygen species (free radicals) which are produced by the body's normal metabolic processes. If they accumulate they can damage key cellular molecules such as DNA and proteins. Cells which do not repair all the damage to DNA may be more prone to developing cancer. Free radicals can also readily oxidise polyunsaturated fatty acids in foods and in cell membranes in the body to give lipid peroxides which can also damage cells. Peroxides, for example those formed by the oxidation of LDL cholesterol (p. 17), may play a part in the formation of the 'plaque' which can build up on the walls of the arteries and eventually cause heart disease (p. 17).

COMA concluded in a report published in 1998, that there was evidence that high intakes of fruit and vegetables were protective against some cancers. However, they also concluded that there is not enough evidence to identify any single component, or mixture of components, as being the active principle, nor that individual vitamins, for example in the form of dietary supplements (vitamin pills) protect against the development of cancers. There is also evidence that high levels of beta-carotene in the form of supplements can actually increase the risk of cancer in people such as smokers who are at high risk. As well as vitamins, fruits and vegetables contain a wide range of other compounds with varying levels of antioxidant activity and it is possible that the range and mix of antioxidant vitamins and other compounds found in fruits and vegetables are necessary for effective protective activity. Research is continuing into the possible role of these compounds in the prevention of heart disease and cancer.

9 Dietary Reference Values for nutrients

An adequate intake of all the essential nutrients is needed for health and activity, and there are additional requirements for growth, pregnancy, lactation and in times of stress such as infection. The exact amounts needed are different for each individual, and depend not only on such readily quantifiable factors as height, weight and sex, but also on physical activity throughout the day, the rate of internal activities such as heartbeat, and the climate.

As these requirements for individuals can only be determined after lengthy experimentation, it is impracticable to determine what they are. Instead, a number of national and international bodies have set standards in the form of recommended nutrient intakes for various groups of the population in question. These recommendations have generally been designed to ensure that the needs of most healthy people will be covered and are therefore higher than estimates of average requirements (except for energy and the energy-yielding constituents). Conversely, the actual nutrient requirements of almost all individuals are less than recommended intakes. Therefore if a person's diet consistently contains more of a nutrient than is recommended, they are almost certainly obtaining more than their requirements. However, if it consistently contains less they could be wrongly diagnosed as deficient, although the further their habitual intake falls below the recommendations, the more likely they are to be malnourished to the extent that they show clinical symptoms. Recommended daily intakes (RDIs) or daily amounts (RDAs) were useful for minimising the risk of dietary deficiency in a population, but they were often used wrongly to assess the adequacy of the diet of an individual when people did not understand how they were derived.

In 1991, the Department of Health published new *Dietary Reference Values* (DRVs), which cover a range of intakes for most nutrients and can therefore be used not only for assessing the adequacy of the diets of groups of people but also, in some circumstances, as a useful reference for those of healthy individuals in the UK. These replace the 1979 RDAs, and there are now three values for most nutrients:

(a) the *Estimated Average Requirement* (EAR). An estimate of the average need for food energy or a nutrient. Many people will need more than this average and many will need less. The EARs for energy in the UK are shown overleaf in Table 24.

67

Table 24. Estimated Average Requirements for energy in the UK (per day).

Age range	Males		Females	
	MJ	kcal	MJ	kcal
0–3 months (formula fed)	2.28	545	2.16	515
4–6 months	2.89	690	2.69	645
7–9 months	3.44	825	3.20	765
10–12 months	3.85	920	3.61	865
1–3 years	5.15	1230	4.86	1165
4–6 years	7.16	1715	6.46	1545
7–10 years	8.24	1970	7.28	1740
11–14 years	9.27	2220	7.92	1845
15–18 years	11.51	2755	8.83	2110
19–50 years	10.60	2550	8.10	1940
51–59 years	10.60	2550	8.00	1900
60–64 years	9.93	2380	7.99	1900
65–74 years	9.71	2330	7.96	1900
75+ years	8.77	2100	7.61	1810
Pregnant			+0.80[a]	+200[a]
Lactating:				
1 month			+1.90	+450
2 months			+2.20	+530
3 months			+2.40	+570
4–6 months			+2.00	+480
>6 months			+1.00	+240

[a] Last trimester only.

(b) the *Reference Nutrient Intake* (RNI), which is the amount of a nutrient that is enough for almost every individual, even those with high needs. The RNI is much higher than most people need and in practice it is very unlikely that anyone consuming this much will be deficient in that nutrient. The RNIs are broadly equivalent to the old RDAs. The RNIs for protein and selected vitamins and minerals are shown in Table 25.

(c) the *Lower Reference Nutrient Intake* (LRNI) is the amount of a nutrient considered to be sufficient only for the small number of individuals with low nutrient needs. Most individuals will need to consume more than this, and people who continually consume less will almost certainly become deficient in that nutrient. Since individual needs vary so widely, DRVs can only provide a guide to the adequacy or otherwise of a diet. Even when intakes are below the LRNI, biochemical measures of adequacy may be needed to determine whether there is really a problem.

As well as those nutrients shown in Table 25, the Department of Health report also gives DRVs for riboflavin, niacin, vitamin B_{12}, vitamin D,

Table 25. Reference Nutrient Intakes for selected nutrients for the UK (per day).

Age range	Protein (g)	Calcium (mg)	Iron (mg)	Zinc (mg)	Vitamin A (µg)	Thiamin (mg)	Vitamin B_6[a] (mg[a])	Folic acid (µg)	Vitamin C (mg)
0–3 months (formula fed)	12.5	525	1.7	4.0	350	0.2	0.2	50	25
4–6 months	12.7	525	4.3	4.0	350	0.2	0.2	50	25
7–9 months	13.7	525	7.8	5.0	350	0.2	0.3	50	25
10–12 months	14.9	525	7.8	5.0	350	0.3	0.4	50	25
1–3 years	14.5	350	6.9	5.0	400	0.5	0.7	70	30
4–6 years	19.7	450	6.1	6.5	500	0.7	0.9	100	30
7–10 years	28.3	550	8.7	7.0	500	0.7	1.0	150	30
Males									
11–14 years	42.1	1000	11.3	9.0	600	0.9	1.2	200	35
15–18 years	55.2	1000	11.3	9.5	700	1.1	1.5	200	40
19–50 years	55.5	700	8.7	9.5	700	1.0	1.4	200	40
50+ years	53.3	700	8.7	9.5	700	0.9	1.4	200	40
Females									
11–14 years	41.2	800	14.8[b]	9.0	600	0.7	1.0	200	35
15–18 years	45.0	800	14.8[b]	7.0	600	0.8	1.2	200	40
19–50 years	45.0	700	14.8[b]	7.0	600	0.8	1.2	200	40
50+ years	46.5	700	8.7	7.0	600	0.8	1.2	200	40
Pregnant	+6.0	c	c	c	+100	+0.1[d]	c	+100	+10
Lactating:									
0–4 months	+11.0	+550	c	+6.0	+350	+0.2	c	+60	+30
over 4 months	+8.0	+550	c	+2.5	+350	+0.2	c	+60	+30

[a] Based on protein providing 14.7 per cent of the EAR for energy.
[b] These RNIs will not meet the needs of approximately 10 per cent of women with the highest menstrual losses, who may need iron supplements.
[c] No increment.
[d] Last trimester only.

phosphorus, magnesium, sodium, potassium, chloride, copper, selenium and iodine.

Additionally, a *safe intake*, in terms of the amount of a nutrient that is enough for almost everyone but below a level which would cause undesirable effects, has been set for each of those nutrients where there was not enough information to estimate DRVs. These include pantothenic acid, biotin, vitamin E, vitamin K, manganese, molybdenum, chromium and fluoride.

For the first time Dietary Reference Values for total fat, fatty acids, starch and sugars, and fibre (as non-starch polysaccharides – NSP) have been produced. Apart from certain fatty acids (see pp. 13–14), none of these nutrients is essential, so that there is no actual requirement for them and EARs could not be set. Instead, desirable population average intakes have been proposed for adults (see Table 26) with a view to improving health and reducing the incidence of diseases such as heart disease and cancer in the UK. The DRVs for fat, carbohydrate and NSP are not intended to be applied to children. Values have not been set for this group because research has not yet established the scientific basis for their needs. It should be noted, however, that children below the age of five, who need energy-dense diets, should not be restricted in their fat intakes.

Table 26. Dietary Reference Values for fat and carbohydrate for adults as percentage of daily energy intake.

	Population average	
	Total energy[a]	Food energy
Saturated fatty acids	10	11
Polyunsaturated fatty acids	6	6.5
Monounsaturated fatty acids	12	13
Trans fatty acids	2	2
Total fat	33	35
Non-milk extrinsic sugars	10	11
Intrinsic and milk sugars, and starch	37	39
Total carbohydrate	47	50
Fibre as non-starch polysaccharides (g/day)	18	18

[a] Includes energy from alcohol

Energy

Appetite normally controls energy intake and keeps it close to requirements. However, this control is not perfect and energy intakes even slightly in excess of requirements are undesirable because they may eventually lead to obesity. Intakes below requirements are also unsatisfactory. The recommendation for each group of people was therefore set at the EAR. Energy needs are found using basal metabolic rates (BMR – see Appendix 2) and physical activity levels (PAL – see p. 25).

$$EAR = BMR \times PAL$$

Although energy is needed during pregnancy for growth of the foetus, placenta and uterus, and for deposition in the mother's body of fat for use during lactation, there is also a reduction in physical activity and metabolic rate. Hence only a modest increase in the EAR for the last three months of pregnancy is recommended. Women who are underweight at the start of pregnancy may need to eat more than this. Energy is also needed for lactation, as breast milk contains enough energy to supply the needs of the growing infant.

Fat

Dietary Reference Values for fatty acids and total fat are given as their percentage contributions to energy intake (Table 26). These should be regarded only as guidelines to desirable intakes, rather than estimates of individual requirements, and are average values for the population consistent with good health; apart from the essential fatty acids (see pp. 13–14), there is no absolute need for these nutrients individually. A breakdown of the different types of fat (e.g. into saturated, unsaturated, etc.) has been included because their varying effects on health (p. 16) are as important to take into account as is total fat intake. The DRV for saturated fatty acids has been set with the intention of reducing the average blood cholesterol level of the population in order to help decrease the incidence of heart disease. To meet this target intake there needs to be a considerable change in people's diets; current recommendations are that present average intakes should be reduced from about 16 per cent to no more than about 10 per cent of dietary energy. Average intakes of polyunsaturated fatty acids (PUFAs) are recommended not to increase and if monounsaturated fatty acid intakes also stay the same, or increase at the expense of PUFAs, total fat intakes must decrease. Total fat intakes are currently recommended to fall to an average of about 35 per cent of dietary energy for the population as a whole.

Carbohydrates

Dietary Reference Values for carbohydrates are also given as their percentage contributions to energy intake. They are expressed in the following terms: non-milk extrinsic (NME) sugars; intrinsic and milk sugars and starch (for definition of terms, see pp. 9–10). Non-milk extrinsic sugars are more detrimental to dental health than other forms of sugar, and it is currently recommended that the target population average intake be about 10 per cent of dietary energy. Starch and intrinsic and milk sugars should therefore provide most of the 50 per cent of dietary energy to be derived from carbohydrate. As the present average intake of NME sugars is about 13 per cent of dietary energy, many people will need to reduce their intakes of certain foods such as table sugar, confectionery, cakes, jam, honey and sugary soft drinks. In practice starch should always provide the major part of the energy intake from carbohydrate.

Average adult intakes of NSP should increase from the present level of 12 g per day to about 18 g per day; more than 32 g daily has no extra benefit. Children should eat proportionately less. Small children under two years of age should not eat fibre-rich foods in place of other energy-rich foods or they may not be able to satisfy their energy needs. The amount of NSP in selected foods is shown in Table 2 (p. 10).

Protein

The DRVs are based on estimates of need. The protein RNIs for adults aged 19 or over are 0.75 g per kg per day. Extra protein is allowed for growth in children, growth of the foetus and maternal tissue in pregnant women, and producing breast milk during lactation. The current average adult protein intake is about 15 per cent of food energy which is above the RNI but not likely to have an adverse effect on health, so it can remain at the present level. Since very high intakes will increase the rate at which kidney function is lost with age, it is recommended that protein intakes should not exceed twice the RNI.

Calcium and zinc

Dietary Reference Values allow for the limited absorption of calcium and zinc from the diet and for the high needs of growing children and adolescents. There is no recommended increase in the intake of calcium for the period of pregnancy as calcium absorption is known to increase during this time, but extra may be needed during lactation to provide for milk production (see Table 25.)

Iron

Values allow for low absorption of iron, but assume that, in general, absorption is about 15 per cent from a mixed diet. Non-haem iron in diets containing no meat is not so well absorbed and habitual vegetarians may need higher iron intakes. The ingestion of foods rich in vitamin C at the same time as non-haem iron sources helps to improve iron absorption. The RNI for women of child-bearing age is much higher than for other groups to take account of blood losses during menstruation, but women with very high menstrual blood losses may need intakes above the RNI. Such women may need to take an iron supplement.

Sodium

The RNI for adults of 1.6 g sodium (about 4 g of salt) is enough to satisfy the physiological needs of almost everyone and there is no advantage in exceeding this value. High intakes of sodium may be associated with high blood pressure. The present average adult intake of about 3.5 g per day (equivalent to about 9 g of salt per day) is considered too high, and current recommendations are that the average population intake of sodium should decrease gradually to about 2.3 g (about 6 g of salt) per day to help decrease the incidence of stroke.

Niacin and vitamin A

Values allow for the contributions made by tryptophan and carotenes to the pre-formed nicotinic acid and retinol intakes respectively. Pregnant women should not take vitamin A supplements (except on medical advice) and should not eat liver or liver products which are extremely rich sources of vitamin A (see p. 52).

Folate

The extra quantity of folic acid/folate required by women who are or may become pregnant, in relation to reducing the risk of neural tube defects in their offspring, is described on p. 60.

Vitamin C

Opinions differ about the quantity of vitamin C required for health. It is generally agreed that 10 mg daily will not only prevent, but also cure, scurvy. The RNI of 40 mg for adults is thought to provide a reasonable safety margin, although smokers may have higher needs (possibly as much as an extra 80 mg per day). The evidence for possible benefits of significantly higher general intakes is still conflicting and studies in this area are continuing.

Vitamin D

For most people in the UK the main source of vitamin D is from the action of sunlight on skin. There are therefore no DRVs for adults of the 18–65 age group. For those confined indoors the RNI is 10 μg per day. Supplementation to 10 μg per day for pregnant and lactating women and to 7 μg per day for infants and children up to 2 years is recommended to overcome seasonal depletion during winter months.

Regulation of nutrient intakes

Excessive intakes of many of the minerals can be harmful, as can excessive intakes of some of the vitamins – especially vitamins A and D which accumulate in the liver. Such intakes are unlikely to arise from food, but may result from the overenthusiastic use of mineral and vitamin supplements. Although our storage capacity for most nutrients apart from energy (as fat) is limited, the healthy body nevertheless contains enough reserves to last for many weeks or months even when there is none in the diet. Thus, while Dietary Reference Values are most conveniently expressed in daily terms, it is not necessary for the diet to contain these quantities *every* day. It is sufficient if the requirements are met *over a period of time*.

Uses of the Dietary Reference Values

ASSESSMENT OF DIETS OF GROUPS OF PEOPLE

For population groups, the EAR for energy and the population averages for fat, carbohydrates and fibre are used. If the average intake of protein, vitamins and minerals of the group is at or above the RNI, there will be very little risk of deficiency within the group. Conversely, the greater the percentage of the population below the RNI, the greater is the risk that deficiencies will occur.

ASSESSMENT OF AN INDIVIDUAL'S DIET

Since most estimates of an individual's nutrient intakes are not very accurate, great care needs to be taken in using DRVs for assessing the adequacy of the diet of an individual. Someone consuming more than the RNI is unlikely to be deficient. Whether a person consuming an intake somewhere between the RNI and the LRNI is getting sufficient will depend on their level of need (high, medium or low), but the closer the intake is to the LRNI the more likely deficiency becomes. However, because people's physiological needs vary considerably, deficiency of a nutrient cannot be diagnosed on the basis of dietary assessment alone.

PLANNING FOOD SUPPLIES FOR LARGE GROUPS

So that everyone in a group (for example in a school or older people's home) gets enough of every nutrient to satisfy their needs, those with high nutrient needs must be catered for. This should be achieved if the food supply provides the RNI.

NUTRITION LABELLING

Special nutrition labelling reference values which have been agreed across the EU are used for this purpose; the UK values do not apply.

PART 2

Nutritional value of food and diets

10 Introduction, and general effects of preparation and processing

Introduction

This part of the manual discusses the nutritional importance of particular foods in the context of the diet as a whole.

The nutritional importance of any food depends upon:

(a) the composition of the raw food or ingredients as grown or purchased
(b) the extent to which its nutrients are lost during storage, processing or cooking, and any addition of nutrients during manufacture
(c) the amount that is usually eaten
(d) each individual's own nutritional needs and the extent to which they have already been met by other foods in the diet.

Many factors combine to produce variations in the nutrient content of foods. *Representative* values for the most important nutrients in a wide selection of foods are given in tables throughout this manual and in Appendix 3, and these should constantly be referred to when using this part of the book. It must be remembered, however, that individual samples or brands may differ considerably from the values quoted. A wider selection of foods and nutrients can be found in the book *The Composition of Foods* (1991), and in its supplements as described on pp. 157–8, for those who wish to estimate their nutrient intakes in more detail.

The general effects of storage, processing and cooking are discussed below, and the application of these principles to specific foods and menus is described in Chapters 11 and 12.

Average nutrient intakes from food consumed at home in Britain during 1997, and the contributions made by major types of food, are shown in Table 27. This table was derived from the National Food Survey, which is a long-running survey conducted by the Department for Environment, Food and Rural Affairs (previously the Ministry of Agriculture, Fisheries and Food), and includes about 6000 representative households throughout Britain each year[1].

Cooking and preservation

Most foods have to be prepared and cooked before they can be eaten. For some foods the process may be simple, as in the peeling of an orange. For

---

[1] From April 2001, data for the National Food Survey have been collected as part of the new Expenditure and Food Survey.

Table 27. Percentage contribution made by groups of foods to the nutrient content of the average household diet in 1997

	Energy	Protein	Fat	Saturated fatty acids	Carbohydrate
Whole Milk	4	5	5	9	2
Other milk and cream	6	10	5	8	5
Cheese	3	5	6	9	0
Total milk, cream, cheese	13	21	17	26	7
Carcase meat	3	10	6	6	0
Other meat and meat products	10	22	16	15	2
Total meat	14	31	22	21	2
Fish	1	5	2	1	0
Eggs	1	3	2	1	0
Fats	10	0	28	22	0
Sugars and preserves	5	0	0	0	10
Potatoes	3	3	0	0	6
Fresh green vegetables	1	1	0	0	1
Other fresh vegetables	1	1	0	0	1
Processed vegetables	5	4	5	5	6
Total vegetables	10	9	6	5	14
Fresh fruit	2	1	0	0	4
Fruit products and nuts	2	1	1	1	3
Total fruit	4	2	2	1	7
Bread	13	14	3	2	21
Flour	1	1	0	0	3
Cakes and biscuits	9	4	9	11	10
Other cereal products	10	7	5	4	16
Total cereals	33	26	17	17	49
Confectionery	2	1	2	3	2
Beverages	0	1	0	0	0
Soft drinks	2	0	0	0	5
Alcoholic drinks	2	0	0	0	0
Total other foods	3	1	3	3	3

Source: Ministry of Agriculture, Fisheries and Food; National Food Survey 1997.
Figures have been rounded to the nearest final digit so there may be an apparent slight discrepancy between the sum of the constituent items and the total shown.
[a] Excludes sodium from table salt

Fibre (NSP)	Calcium	Iron	Sodium[a]	Vitamin C	Vitamin A retinol equivalent	Thiamin
0	15	1	2	3	4	2
0	29	1	4	6	7	5
0	11	0	4	0	6	0
0	55	2	9	9	17	7
0	0	4	1	0	0	4
2	3	10	20	3	22	11
2	3	14	21	3	22	15
0	2	2	3	0	0	1
0	1	2	1	0	3	1
0	1	0	5	0	22	0
0	0	1	0	1	0	0
8	0	3	0	9	0	8
4	2	3	0	7	2	3
7	1	3	0	8	21	3
19	3	8	9	9	5	5
38	6	17	9	32	29	19
9	1	2	0	21	1	2
2	1	2	0	24	0	3
11	2	4	1	45	1	5
20	14	21	24	0	0	20
2	2	1	0	0	0	2
5	4	7	5	0	1	3
18	4	21	9	2	1	19
45	24	51	38	2	3	43
0	1	1	0	0	0	0
0	1	2	0	0	0	1
0	1	0	1	7	1	0
0	1	1	0	0	0	0
2	2	3	11	1	1	7

others it may be complicated: for example, wheat grains must be separated from the inedible parts of the plant and milled into flour, which in turn may need to be treated before being baked into bread. At each stage, some of the nutrients will be discarded or destroyed, whether the process takes place in a factory or in the home. The nutrients may be further reduced if the food is stored for long periods, particularly if conditions are not ideal.

Although these losses are usually not of major significance if a good mixed diet is eaten (as this will still provide a considerable excess of nutrients over the Reference Nutrient Intakes), it is nevertheless desirable that the losses are kept to a minimum. A discussion of the main methods of cooking and preserving foods is therefore followed by descriptions of the factors which tend to reduce the stability of each nutrient. Applications to specific foods are discussed in Chapter 11.

COOKING

Heat is generally applied to food in one of three ways:
(a) directly, with or without additional fat – as in roasting, grilling and baking (120–250°C; 250–475°F), and microwave cooking.
(b) with water – as in boiling, stewing and braising (100°C; 212°F).
(c) with fat – frying (155–225°C; 310–435°F).

Heat causes chemical and physical changes in food which in general make the flavour, palatability and digestibility of the raw product more acceptable and may improve its keeping quality. Heat may also increase the availability of some nutrients by destroying enzymes and anti-digestive factors. But cooking more usually results in the loss of nutrients, this being greatest at high temperatures with long cooking times, or if an excessive amount of liquid is used. The losses of soluble vitamins and minerals are, of course, reduced if meat juices and cooking water are not discarded but used in (for example) soups or gravies.

The effects of microwaves and infra-red cooking on nutrients are similar to the effects of the more traditional methods they replace. When used for reheating, they cause little additional destruction of nutrients.

FREEZING

This popular method of food preservation may result in some loss of thiamin and vitamin C when vegetables are blanched in water before freezing, but less than would otherwise result from the continuing action of enzymes in the plant tissues during storage. If the frozen foods are kept below −18°C (0°F) for a year there is little further loss of nutritional value until the food is thawed. In general, differences between the nutrient content of cooked fresh foods and cooked frozen foods as served on the plate are small.

Processing in a factory is mainly intended to preserve food so that the choice is greater and independent of geographical area or the season of the year, and to reduce the time spent on preparing food in the home. The main commercial processes which cause some loss of nutrients are blanching, heat processing, and drying or dehydration.

Blanching or scalding in water or steam is done mainly to minimise enzyme activity, and is a first step in the preservation of most vegetables for subsequent freezing, canning or dehydration. The process is usually carefully controlled, but small amounts of some minerals and water-soluble vitamins dissolve in the water or steam and are lost.

Freezing itself has little effect on nutritional value, and since the delay after harvesting is minimal the nutrients in the high-quality fresh foods that are used are generally well retained.

Heat processing in metal cans or bottling in glass jars will reduce the amounts of heat-sensitive vitamins, especially thiamin, folate and vitamin C. The losses will depend on the length of time needed to destroy any harmful organisms and to cook the food, and will be greater for larger cans and in foods of a solid consistency, such as ham, because of the slow transfer of heat from the outside to the centre. They will also depend on the acidity of the food and the presence of light and air, so that it is difficult to give precise values for expected losses.

Dehydration (in air) in carefully controlled conditions has little effect on most nutrients, but destroys about half the vitamin C. Thiamin is completely lost if sulphur dioxide is added as a preservative. Prolonged sun drying as in the production of raisins allows substantial changes to occur. Suitable packaging of dried foods is essential to prevent nutrient losses during their prolonged storage life.

Stability of individual nutrients

PROTEIN

Protein is denatured by heat, and when cooking conditions are severe it becomes less available for utilisation within the body. This is partly because the changes in structure make the protein more difficult to digest and partly because some of the component amino acids are destroyed – most notably lysine, which can react with carbohydrates in the food. These losses can also occur during prolonged storage even at room temperature.

VITAMIN A

Both retinol and beta-carotene are stable throughout most cooking procedures, although at high temperatures and in the presence of air (e.g. when butter or margarine are used in frying or when vegetables are canned) there will be some loss. Some loss also occurs during prolonged storage if light and air are not rigorously excluded.

B-VITAMINS

The *B-vitamins* are all water-soluble and most are also sensitive to heat.

Thiamin is one of the least stable of vitamins. It is readily dissolved out of foods into the cooking water and is easily lost in the juices from meat. It is fairly stable to heat if the food is acid, but the losses can be considerable under alkaline conditions, especially if sodium bicarbonate is added during cooking. It has been calculated that on average about 20 per cent of the thiamin content of all the food brought into the home is lost during cooking and reheating, but the loss is greater in some foods than in others. Any foods which have been preserved by the use of sulphur dioxide, such as sausages, wine and some potato products, will contain very little thiamin.

Riboflavin can be lost in discarded cooking water and meat juices; it is also unstable to alkali, and especially sensitive to light.

Niacin is an exceptionally stable vitamin, and will be lost only through its solubility in water.

Other B-vitamins are all soluble in water. Vitamin B_6, folate and pantothenic acid are also sensitive to heat, and can therefore be lost in cooking and canning.

VITAMIN C

Vitamin C is perhaps the least stable of all the vitamins. In addition to being water-soluble, it is very readily destroyed by air. This destruction is accelerated by heat, by alkali, and by the presence of certain metals, e.g. copper or iron. Vitamin C is also rapidly oxidised when an enzyme present in fruit and vegetables is released by any physical damage to the plant such as cutting. Thus poor cooking practices such as prolonged boiling of green vegetables in large amounts of water containing sodium bicarbonate to improve the colour, followed by keeping them hot, can result in destruction of all the vitamin C originally present. Vitamin C is, however, partly protected by sulphur dioxide.

OTHER VITAMINS AND MINERALS

Vitamin D is stable to normal cooking procedures.

Vitamin E is not soluble in water and is stable to heat. It is, however, oxidised in the presence of air.

Minerals are unaffected by heat processing, but can be lost by leaching into water during moist cooking or processing.

Table 28 summarises the sensitivity of the most important nutrients.

Table 28. Summary of factors (✓) which may reduce the nutrients in food.

Nutrient	Heat	Light	Air	Water (by leaching)	Acid	Alkali	Other
Protein	✓ if prolonged						
Minerals				✓			
Vitamin A	✓ with air		✓ with heat				Metals
Thiamin[a]	✓		✓	✓		✓	Sulphur dioxide
Riboflavin		✓		✓		✓	
Folate	✓		✓ (but protected by vitamin C)	✓		✓	
Vitamin C[a]	✓	✓	✓ (but protected by sulphur dioxide)	✓		✓	Enzymes; metals

[a] Least stable to cooking and storage.

11   Foods

Milk

IMPORTANCE IN THE DIET

Cow's milk is the most complete of all foods, containing nearly all the constituents of nutritional importance to humans; it is, however, comparatively deficient in iron and vitamins C and D. Unlike other foods of animal origin, milk contains a significant amount of carbohydrate, in the form of the disaccharide lactose (p. 6).

Typical amounts of the major nutrients present in 1 pint (568 ml) of whole milk and of skimmed and semi-skimmed milks are given in Table 29. Milk from the Jersey and Guernsey breeds of cow contains rather more fat than milk from other breeds (1 pint providing 26.7 g fat) as well as more beta-carotene and calcium.

Table 29. Nutrients per pint in various types of cow's milk.

	Whole	Semi-skimmed	Skimmed
Energy (kJ)	1611	1148	822
(kcal)	385	272	193
Protein (g)	18.7	19.4	19.4
Fat (g)	22.8	9.4	0.6
Carbohydrate (g)	28.1	29.4	29.4
Calcium (mg)	673	705	706
Iron (mg)	0.3	0.3	0.3
Sodium (mg)	322	323	318
Vitamin A (retinol equivalent) (µg)	325	132	6
Thiamin (mg)	0.17	0.23	0.23
Riboflavin (mg)	0.99	1.06	1
Niacin equivalent (mg)	4.7	5.3	5.3
Vitamin B_{12} (µg)	2.3	2.3	2.4
Vitamin C (mg)	6	6	6
Vitamin D (µg)	0.17	0.06	0

Values decline on storage in the home.

Average milk consumption is now just under half a pint (264 ml) per day, sixty per cent of which is reduced-fat milk (skimmed and semi-skimmed milk).

84

The contribution which these various types of milk make to the nutrient content of the average household diet is shown in Table 27. It can be seen that in a mixed diet milk is particularly valuable for its content of high-quality protein and easily assimilated calcium, and as a rich source of riboflavin; moreover, milk provides good nutritional value for money (pp. 112–13).

Unmodified cow's milk is not suitable for infants under one year of age as their main drink because it doesn't contain enough iron and other nutrients. It is important that young children are given concentrated sources of energy. Thus whole milk, not reduced-fat milks, should be given to children between the ages of one and two years. Those over two but under five can be given semi-skimmed, but not skimmed milk. Reduced-fat milks are, however, useful for adults who drink a lot of milk and who wish to reduce their fat intake (p. 116).

It is important that bottled milks are not left on the doorstep exposed directly to sunlight for more than an hour, since a substantial amount of the riboflavin and vitamin C can be destroyed.

EFFECTS OF COOKING

The bubbles of steam formed as milk is heated are stabilised by the protein and this gives rise to the characteristic 'boiling over'. Food such as fish or vegetables, when baked in the milk, can cause coagulation of milk proteins, but this does not affect their digestibility. Some caramelisation of the sugars in milk may occur with long cooking in a very slow oven, as for example in milk puddings or in the production of sterilised or evaporated milk.

EFFECTS OF PROCESSING

When milk is *homogenised* the fat globules are broken up mechanically and distributed throughout the milk so that they no longer rise to form a creamy layer at the top of the milk bottle. The nutritional value of homogenised milk is similar to that of pasteurised whole milk.

Skimmed milk has almost all of its fat removed, and *semi-skimmed milk* must by law contain only between 1.5 and 1.8 per cent fat. The fat-soluble vitamins A and D are reduced proportionately (only traces remain in skimmed milk), but the calcium content remains almost unchanged (see Table 29). *Dried skimmed milk*, and similar products with added vegetable fat, may be fortified with vitamins A and D.

A variety of heat treatments can be used to improve the keeping quality of liquid milk. The fat, fat-soluble vitamins, carbohydrates and minerals of milk are not affected by heat, but when the heat treatment is relatively harsh slight changes occur in the availability of some of the amino acids in the milk proteins. The vitamins in milk which are partially destroyed by heat processing are vitamin C, thiamin, pyridoxine, vitamin B_{12} and folate.

Most of the liquid milk supply in the UK is pasteurised. During this relatively mild form of heat treatment the milk is heated to 72°C (162°F) for 15 seconds, killing any disease-causing bacteria. About 10 per cent of the thiamin and vitamin B_{12}, and 25 per cent of the vitamin C are destroyed, but in a mixed diet milk is not an important source of these nutrients. The ultra-high temperature (UHT) treatment of milk, in which a temperature of about 135°C (275°F) is maintained for at least one second, also causes some vitamin losses which are very similar to the losses in pasteurisation. UHT or 'long-life' milk is packed aseptically into special containers which protect it from light and from oxygen. It will keep satisfactorily for several months without refrigeration, but variable losses of vitamin C and folate may occur during prolonged storage. Once opened, however, UHT milk is as perishable as fresh milk.

Sterilised milk is subjected to a more drastic form of heat treatment; it is prepared from homogenised milk which is usually bottled and then heated to about 110°C (230°F) for 20–30 minutes. About 60 per cent of the vitamin C in the raw milk and 20 per cent of the thiamin are destroyed during the process.

Evaporated milk is prepared by the concentration of liquid milk at low temperatures; the milk is subsequently sterilised in cans at, for example, 115°C (239°F) for 15 minutes. In general, the nutrient losses are similar to those in sterilised milk.

Sweetened condensed milk is prepared similarly to evaporated milk, but since it contains added sucrose the processing temperature needed for an adequate storage life is lower. Nutrient losses are therefore lower too, and are generally similar to those that occur in pasteurisation.

Milk products

CHEESE

When rennet is added to warm acidified milk, the milk protein casein coagulates to form a firm curd which is treated in various ways to make cheeses of different kinds. Most of the protein, fat and vitamin A and much of the calcium in the milk remain in the curd, while a large part of the lactose and B-vitamins are lost with the whey as it drains away. Further minor changes in vitamin content occur during ripening and storage – processes which are greatly affected by the amount of salt present. Cheddar cheese consists very roughly of one-third protein, one-third fat and one-third water. Although methods of preparation differ, the amounts of protein and fat in whole-milk cheeses are fairly similar. Reduced-fat versions of Cheddar and some other cheeses are now available. *Hard cheeses*, such as Cheddar and Double Gloucester, in general contain more nutrients per 100 g than *soft cheeses*, such as Camembert, because they contain less moisture. Some cheeses are not ripened, such as cottage cheese, cream cheese, fromage frais and quark. *Fromage frais* is a very soft cheese with a mild and fresh taste. Although its fat content varies according to the starting material, most products sold have a relatively low fat content compared to hard and soft cheeses. *Cottage cheese* is made from skimmed milk and therefore contains very little fat; *cream cheese* has a high fat content. Certain cheeses are made from milk other than cow's milk; for example *feta cheese* is traditionally made from goat's or sheep's milk.

YOGURT

The nutritional value of yogurt is similar to that of the milk and minor ingredients used in its preparation, except that in products with added sugar or added fat the energy content is increased. Most commercial yogurts are based either on whole milk or on skimmed milk which is inoculated with a selected culture of lactic bacteria under controlled conditions. Dried skimmed milk, pectin or modified starch may be added to produce a firmer or more 'creamy' consistency; flavourings, fruit juices, fruit, nuts and sugar or non-sugar sweeteners are often incorporated to give a varied product. Some varieties of yogurt are fortified with vitamins A and D. Depending on the type of milk from which it is made, the fat content of yogurt can vary from about 0.2 g per 100 g in low-calorie yogurt to about 9 g per 100 g in Greek yogurt made with cow's milk.

ICE CREAM

The nutrient composition of dairy ice cream varies with the amounts of sugar, milk, dried milk, butterfat and cream which it contains. It can make a useful contribution to the daily intake of energy and calcium, particularly for people who have small appetites or who will not drink milk. Although most ice cream in the UK is based on skimmed milk with non-dairy fats instead of, or as well as milk fat, it is still a good source of calcium. Sorbets (water ices) are not based on milk, but consist of a mixture of water, fruit and variable amounts of added sugar.

BUTTER

Butter is made by churning cream in a rotating drum so that the fat globules separate from the liquid buttermilk. In England and Wales butter must contain not less than 80 per cent milk fat, not more than 2 per cent milk solids other than fat and not more than 16 per cent water. During manufacture, 1–2 per cent of salt is added to salted butter. The amounts of vitamins A and D in butter vary; representative values are shown in Appendix 3. *Ghee* is made by the prolonged heating of butter. The emulsion breaks down and on cooling the pure fat can be separated from the water so that ghee contains virtually no water. Vegetable ghee, made from vegetable oil, can also be obtained.

Cream is derived from fresh milk either by skimming off the fatty layer which rises to the surface or in a mechanical separator. Minimum fat contents for different types of cream are specified in Government Regulations; these include: half cream, 12 per cent by weight as milk fat; single cream, 18 per cent; whipping cream 35 per cent; double cream 48 per cent; and clotted cream, 55 per cent fat. These compare with an average of 3.9 per cent fat in whole milk. The energy value of different types of cream varies directly with the fat content. Sour cream is made by adding a bacterial culture to the cream to slightly sour it and give it a thicker consistency. Sour cream is nutritionally similar to the cream from which it is made.

Meat

The average nutrient composition of various types of meat is shown in Appendix 3. Genetic breeding and changes in methods of animal husbandry have resulted in leaner meat, particularly in the case of sheep and pigs, than that of a decade ago. More of the external fat may also be trimmed off prior to sale.

Muscle tissue is composed of bundles of muscle fibres surrounded by connective tissue and associated with intramuscular fat. Each separate muscle fibre is a tube composed largely of water, and containing soluble proteins, mineral salts, vitamins and flavours. The eating quality of meat is largely determined by the relative proportions of connective tissue and muscle fibres in a particular cut and the amount of 'marbling' fat that is present within the lean, but the overall nutrient content of lean meat from the more expensive cuts is not significantly different from that in other parts of the carcase.

IMPORTANCE IN THE DIET

Meat is a good source of high-quality protein, of available iron and zinc, and of all the B-vitamins except folate. Pork, bacon and ham in particular are rich in thiamin. Liver, and to a lesser extent, kidney, are also rich in vitamin A and folate (thus differing from carcase meat) and in iron, riboflavin and other B-vitamins. Sweetbreads and tripe are useful and easily digestible sources of animal protein. Tripe also contains more calcium than other meats; this is derived from the lime with which it is treated during preparation. Liver and kidney and chicken and turkey meat (especially if the skin is removed) contain less fat than most carcase meat and their energy content is therefore lower. Much of the fat can nevertheless be trimmed from beef, lamb and pork before or after cooking. Mince may be heated and the melted fat poured off before further cooking takes place.

Consumption of poultry meat is about 15 times higher than it was in 1955, and is greater than the consumption of beef. This trend is due to the growth of the broiler industry and the consequent fall in the price of poultry. Small differences in the nutrient composition of broiler chickens and free-range chickens are of no significance in a mixed diet.

EFFECTS OF COOKING

The muscle protein myoglobin which provides the red colour of raw meat is changed by heat, and the brown colour associated with cooked meat develops at temperatures above 65°C. Heat causes the proteins in the muscle fibres to coagulate and the meat becomes firm; shrinkage occurs and this in turn causes extrusion of meat juices and a loss of weight. Losses of fat and meat juices increase as the temperature rises, so the total weight loss is influenced by the cooking temperature and the internal temperature which the meat reaches as well as by the cooking time; thus the effects of grilling and frying are similar. The substantial variations that occur in the proportions of bone, muscle and fat in different parts of different carcases also affect the nutrients that are actually available from a given weight of fresh meat. It is thus very important, when estimating the contributions made by meat to the nutrient content of a diet, to weigh each cut after cooking and removal of any fat or bone.

Some cheaper cuts of meat which contain a higher proportion of connective tissue are more palatable if a slow moist method of cooking, such as stewing or braising, is used for the preparation; this allows the collagen in the connective tissue to be converted to gelatin thus making the meat more tender. Pressure cooking is also useful for this purpose.

Cooking does not affect the minerals present in meat but a proportion of those which are soluble pass into the exuded juices or dissolve in the cooking water. Similarly, since the B-vitamins are all water-soluble, varying amounts will be found in the drip, meat juice and stock. Losses of B-vitamins from fried or grilled meat are around 20 per cent. Destruction of thiamin, niacin, pyridoxine and pantothenic acid in stewed meat varies between 30 and 70 per cent, although overall losses are smaller if the gravy or liquid from a stew is consumed. About 30 per cent of the folate is lost from stewed liver and kidney. After cooking, there are only small differences in the content of the B-vitamins in fresh and frozen meat. Vitamin A is relatively stable to heat, and is not affected by most cooking procedures, although some loss occurs during frying at high temperatures (above 200°C).

There is no evidence of any significant loss of nutrients from meat during freezing, but the drip which collects on thawing will contain some soluble nutrients.

Meat juices are water-soluble substances from meat which include peptides, B-vitamins and mineral salts. They provide, with fat, most of the flavour and aroma of meat and act as a stimulant to appetite and to the secretion of gastric juice.

Stock can be made by boiling meat bones in water. The hot water extracts a small amount of fat and gelatin from the bone marrow together with other minor components which provide the flavour. Stock is usually used as a basis for soup and it is the addition of other ingredients (e.g. milk, fat and flour in cream soups) which provides most of the nutritional value of the soup.

Meat products

The meat content of meat products such as sausages is controlled by Government Regulations (p. 155). The important contribution which meat products make to the nutrient content of the average household diet is shown on p. 78; average consumption per head is now rather greater than for carcase meat.

The most usual methods of heat treatment before any domestic cooking are roasting, baking and canning, all of which cause some loss of thiamin and a slight reduction in the quality of the meat protein. The loss of thiamin when meat is canned is generally slightly greater than in cooked meat. Corned beef is prepared from cured meat which is trimmed, coarsely cut and cooked before canning; after this process very little thiamin remains in the finished product. Commercial *meat extract* is a by-product of the meat industry. The liquid in which meat and bone have been heated is concentrated after the removal of some of the fat. Such products, including stock cubes, are also rich in sodium. When the meat extract containing the dissolved solids is diluted again for consumption, the amount of protein and energy which it contributes to the soup or beverage is too small to be of importance in the diet; nevertheless it contains minerals besides the salt and vitamins, and is a useful stimulant to appetite.

The nutrient losses that occur during the cooking of meat products are similar to those that occur during the cooking of carcase meat.

Fish

IMPORTANCE IN THE DIET

The flesh or muscle of fish is a valuable source of protein which is of a similar quality to that of meat and milk. It can be seen from Appendix 3 that the amount of fat in different kinds of fish varies widely; the flesh of white fish, such as cod, haddock, plaice and whiting, contains very little fat (1–2 per cent) while that of fatty fish (herring, mackerel, trout, salmon, eel) varies from about 5 per cent to more than 20 per cent. There can also be considerable variation within one type of fatty fish, depending on the season of the year or the level of maturity attained by the fish. In general, the vitamin content of white fish muscle is similar to that of lean meat. The fat-soluble vitamins A and D are present in the flesh of fatty fish and in the livers of fish such as cod and halibut. Oils from the latter may therefore be used as concentrated vitamin supplements. Fish oils also contain long-chain *n-3* polyunsaturated fatty acids which may play a favourable role in helping to prevent coronary heart disease (see p. 17). Fish muscle contains a well-balanced supply of minerals including iodine, and if the bones are eaten, as for example in sardines and canned salmon, these are a good source of calcium, phosphorus and fluoride.

EFFECTS OF COOKING AND PROCESSING

The changes that occur when fish is cooked are similar to those in meat but the shrinkage is not so great; losses of mineral salts are proportional to the loss of water. The vitamin A and vitamin D in fatty fish are both heat-stable. Canned tuna is a poor source of the long-chain *n-3* polyunsaturated fatty acids as processing reduces the fat content of the fish to a low level. Canning of other fatty fish has little effect on their fat content, so that canned sardines, pilchards and salmon remain good sources of *n-3* polyunsaturated fatty acids. When fish is canned or cured by smoking there is some loss of thiamin, but otherwise these processes have little effect on the nutrients in fish. Modern methods of freezing do not affect the nutritive value, and poaching and steaming incur only small losses of vitamins. Between 10 and 30 per cent losses of B-vitamins occur on baking, frying or grilling. For estimating the cooked weight of fish, a loss of about 15 per cent may be assumed on gentle cooking unless frying is used: fish fried in batter and fish products which are fried will gain fat on cooking.

Eggs

IMPORTANCE IN THE DIET

The consumption of eggs has decreased significantly over the last 20 years, but eggs can still make a small but useful contribution to the daily intakes of vitamin D, retinol, riboflavin, iodine and protein in the average diet and for the elderly they can be an important source of protein, vitamin B_{12} and vitamin D. It used to be thought that eggs were a good source of iron; however, it is now known that the form in which iron occurs in egg yolk is not easily absorbed by the body.

The shell colour is related to the breed of hen rather than to nutrient content and in this respect it is therefore unimportant; similarly a deep-yellow yolk does not necessarily indicate a high vitamin A content since the pigment is not beta-carotene.

It has been shown that there is no practical difference in the composition of eggs obtained from battery, deep-litter and free-range hens.

EFFECTS OF COOKING

When eggs are boiled or fried the proteins coagulate first in the white, at approximately 60°C (140°F), then in the yolk. This property makes eggs suitable for binding dry ingredients together in cooking, and for thickening sauces and soups; the mixture of eggs and milk sets in baked egg custard. Over-cooking causes the proteins to curdle and contract slightly and a yellow watery fluid to separate out; this may occur when scrambling eggs or boiling sauces to which eggs have been added.

The black discoloration which is sometimes present around the yolk of hard-boiled eggs is iron sulphide. This is formed during cooking from hydrogen sulphide in the egg white and iron in the egg yolk. The blackening can be reduced by cooling the eggs in water immediately after cooking.

When egg whites are beaten, the proteins hold air to form a stable foam which coagulates or sets at a very low temperature, as in meringues. Eggs are also used for aeration, for example in sponge cakes, and to promote the emulsification of fat, as in mayonnaise. Some of the heat-sensitive B-vitamins are lost during cooking. For example, the average loss of thiamin which results from boiling, frying, poaching and scrambling is between 5 and 15 per cent; similar losses of niacin also occur and slightly higher losses (15–30 per cent) of these and other B-vitamins take place in baked dishes. During frying, the fat content of eggs may be increased by about 50 per cent.

Pulses, nuts and seeds

Pulses or legumes such as dried peas, beans, chickpeas and lentils, and the range of canned pulse products now available, are rich in protein and are an excellent source of fibre. In general they are used as meat alternatives, especially by vegetarians and vegans. They provide more energy and B-vitamins than many vegetables, but do not contain vitamin C. Baked beans are often eaten as a vegetable, and a beverage (previously known as soya milk) derived from soya beans is used as an animal milk substitute and is sometimes fortified with calcium and sweetened with fruit juice. Soya flour and other products derived from soya are increasingly used in manufactured foods. They are nutritionally valuable, but extra nutrients are added if they are intended to resemble or replace meat (see p. 21).

Nuts, peanuts (which are actually a type of legume) and derived products such as peanut butter are rich in fat and are consequently a concentrated source of energy. They are an excellent source of protein and fibre and a good source of B-vitamins and vitamin E, but contain no vitamin A or C.

Seeds from sunflowers, pumpkins and sesame, and products such as tahini paste from sesame seeds, have a nutritional value similar to nuts.

Cereals

IMPORTANCE IN THE DIET

Cereal grains are a major component of the human diet throughout the world. In Britain, wheat in the form of bread, flour, biscuits, cakes and pasta, together with other cereals such as rice, oatmeal and breakfast cereals, provides about one-third of the total energy, a quarter of the protein and about half of the carbohydrate, fibre and iron in the average household diet, although the iron is poorly absorbed. Cereals also make a substantial contribution to the intake of many other nutrients, particularly calcium, niacin and thiamin which are added to most flours, sodium from added salt, and fibre. In general, the common cereals (wheat, oats, barley, rye, maize and rice) contain 65–80 per cent carbohydrate (starch), 7–13 per cent protein, 1–9 per cent fat, 2–15 per cent fibre and approximately 12 per cent moisture in the whole grain. Advances in plant breeding have led to the development of cereal varieties which are richer in lysine; some increases in protein levels may be obtained experimentally by the appropriate use of manures and fertilisers.

NUTRIENT LOSSES IN MILLING AND THE COMPOSITION OF FLOUR

The distribution of nutrients within the wheat grain is not uniform. The concentration of protein, minerals and vitamins is higher in the germ and outer layers of the grain than in the inner starchy endosperm; thus when wheat is milled to produce white flour a proportion of the nutrients and fibre is discarded with the bran and germ. Owing to the continuing, if decreasing, preference for white flour in the British diet, those nutrients lost in the refining process which are of importance in relation to the diet as a whole are replaced. Similar losses of minerals and vitamins occur in the milling of rice unless it is parboiled, a process which causes nutrients to migrate from the outer to the inner parts of the grain.

The composition of flour in the UK is controlled by Government Regulations (p. 153-4) which require that all flours contain minimum quantities of two B-vitamins (thiamin and niacin) and iron which correspond to the levels occurring naturally in 80 per cent extraction flour[1]. These quantities are listed overleaf.

---

[1] The weight of flour obtained from a given weight of cleaned grain, expressed as a percentage, is known as the *extraction rate*.

	per 100 g
Iron	1.65 mg
Thiamin (vitamin B_1)	0.24 mg
Niacin	1.60 mg

White flours of about 73 per cent extraction, as used now, have to be fortified with these nutrients to bring their concentrations to the prescribed levels; wholemeal flours contain more than the specified minimum quantities. In addition calcium carbonate must be added to all flours except wholemeal and certain self-raising flours at the rate of 235–390 mg per 100 g.

WHOLEMEAL, BROWN AND WHITE FLOURS

The composition of each of these flours varies, but in general wholemeal flour contains somewhat greater amounts of most minerals and several vitamins, particularly of the B group, but less calcium than the flours to which calcium has been added. Wholemeal flour also contains more fibre and phytic acid than brown or white flour. However, apart from the fibre content, nutritional differences between wholemeal and the fortified brown and white flours are unlikely to be of practical significance in a mixed diet.

Flours which will produce a large loaf of good quality need to contain sufficient gluten, either from 'strong' varieties of wheat or else added separately. 'Weak' wheats give flours which are more suitable for making biscuits and cakes.

EFFECTS OF COOKING AND PROCESSING

Cooking causes the starch granules of which cereal carbohydrate is composed to swell and gelatinise, thus making the starch digestible (p. 7); it also results in a tripling (approximately) of the weight of rice and pasta on boiling as they take up water.

Thiamin is the vitamin mainly affected during the baking or processing of cereal products because it is sensitive to heat and destroyed by alkali. The amount lost therefore varies with the cooking time and the final temperature of the cooked food, and whether or not baking powder is used, as for example in soda bread or scones. Riboflavin and niacin are more stable to heat and the loss on baking is small. Of the other unstable vitamins, folate is low in wheat, and vitamin C is only present if added as a flour improver before making bread. It is then destroyed on baking.

In bread-making the yeast gradually ferments the sugars which are formed from the starch in the dough, breaking them down to alcohol and then to carbon dioxide and water, much of which is driven off. The carbon dioxide causes the bread to rise. When water is added to the flour in the preparation of the dough the proteins gliadin and glutenin combine to form gluten. During baking, the yeast is killed and fermentation ceases. The gluten holds the pockets of gas and then coagulates as cooking proceeds, holding the bread in shape. The gelatinised starch in the bread also contributes to loaf structure. The average loss of thiamin in baking bread is about 15 per cent.

About 80 per cent of the bread sold in the UK is made by the *Chorleywood Bread Process* in which addition of certain substances (improvers) to the mix, and the replacement of conventional fermentation of the dough by a few minutes of intense mechanical agitation in special high speed mixers, decreases production time and allows UK and European wheats to be used. It has been shown that breads produced by this process do not differ significantly in nutritional value from those made by conventional methods.

Toast

When bread is toasted the thiamin content is further reduced; the total loss on toasting is about 15 per cent. The heat drives off water from the bread, so that the content of energy and most other nutrients per unit weight increases or remains the same.

Cakes and biscuits

When making a cake, such as a Victoria sponge cake, air is introduced into the mixture by creaming together the fat and sugar. The eggs are lightly beaten to incorporate air before being added to the creamed mixture and the flour is folded in lightly so that this air is not forced out. During cooking the starch gelatinises and the flour and egg proteins coagulate. The loss of thiamin when making cakes and biscuits varies between 20 and 30 per cent.

The relative proportions of fat and sugar to flour and other ingredients are important in giving different cakes and biscuits their characteristic textures and tastes.

Breakfast cereals

The heat treatment used in the preparation of breakfast cereals destroys a large proportion of the thiamin present in the whole grain. In puffed and flaked products it is usually a total loss but the process used in the preparation of shredded wheat is less drastic and only about half the thiamin is destroyed. Many breakfast cereals are therefore enriched with thiamin, as well as a wide range of other vitamins including folic acid and vitamin B_{12}, and iron. Sugar, salt and bran are also added to many products, which are an important source of nutrients for many people. Muesli and some other cereal products also have a variety of dried fruits and nuts added. These, and bran-enriched products, provide an excellent source of fibre. Some types of processing lead to an increase in the proportion of starch that is resistant to digestion (see p. 7) and which may have some functions similar to fibre. When porridge is made from coarse oatmeal the cooking loss of thiamin is about 10 per cent.

Roots, tubers and plantains

POTATOES

Importance in the diet

In many diets potatoes provide the main source of vitamin C, even though the vitamin content per unit weight is comparatively low. The amount is highest in new potatoes and falls gradually during post-harvest storage. Instant potato powder and potato flakes or granules are nutritionally equivalent alternatives to fresh potatoes only if the vitamin C and thiamin which are lost in processing are added back to the products. Because of the comparatively large amounts which are eaten, potatoes contribute more protein and iron than other vegetables in the average diet and they are also useful sources of thiamin, niacin and several other nutrients including fibre.

Effects of cooking

The digestibility of raw potato starch is very poor, but is greatly improved by cooking. Careless peeling of potatoes which removes a significant proportion of the flesh along with the skin can result in the loss of vitamin C and some minerals. Water-soluble vitamins and some minerals are lost more readily from peeled potatoes than from potatoes cooked in their skins. Average losses of vitamin C from potatoes are:

Method of cooking potatoes	Vitamin C lost (%)
Boiled after peeling	20–50
Boiled in their skins	20–40
Baked in their skins	10–40
Roasted	15–50
Chipped or fried	15–30

If cooked potatoes are mashed and then kept hot, the loss of vitamin C is greater than if they are left whole under similar conditions.

Potato whiteners or sulphite dips prevent the discoloration of raw pre-peeled potatoes when they are prepared centrally for distribution to restaurants and other catering establishments, but the amount of thiamin which is lost when the treated potatoes are boiled or fried as chips and subsequently kept hot is greatly increased by this treatment.

The fat content of chips varies from less than 5 per cent of their weight in oven chips to more than 20 per cent in fine-cut French fries. In home-prepared or retail chips, it is lowest when the chips are cut large to reduce their surface area, and when the frying oil is kept hot. Fat content can also be reduced by draining the chips on absorbent paper before serving. The amount of the different fatty acids they or other fried vegetables contain depends on the oil or fat in which they have been fried.

TROPICAL STAPLES

In the UK, cassava and sweetpotatoes (roots) and yams and eddoes (tubers) are at present eaten in quantity mainly in the ethnic communities particularly by those people originating in Asia, Africa and the West Indies. Plantains (green bananas) are not roots, but fruits. However they occupy a similar place in the diet of communities from Africa and the West Indies. Like potatoes, these foods provide moderate amounts of energy, fibre, vitamins and minerals. Cassava and sweetpotato are similar to potatoes in their vitamin C content, and orange-fleshed, but not white-fleshed, sweetpotatoes can contain substantial quantities of beta-carotene.

Vegetables

IMPORTANCE IN THE DIET

Although they contain 80–95 per cent of water, vegetables supply appreciable quantities of nutrients in the average diet. They are also an important source of fibre (p. 7). Many people do not eat nearly enough vegetables, but their range of colours and textures can be exploited to prepare attractive, appetizing and healthy meals. The composition of different vegetables is given in Appendix 3. Their nutrient content is influenced by a number of factors during growth and after harvesting and different samples of the same vegetable can vary considerably. For example, the amount of vitamin C will vary with variety, maturity and exposure to sunlight, as well as with the method of handling, the temperature during transport and the delay before the 'fresh' produce is eaten.

GREEN AND SALAD VEGETABLES

Green vegetables, and salad items such as green peppers and tomatoes, are of nutritional importance because of their contribution to the daily intake of vitamin C, beta-carotene (which after absorption is converted to vitamin A in the body), folate, iron and other minerals, and fibre. They are especially valuable when eaten raw, as they will suffer no cooking losses; there will, however, be considerable losses of vitamin C and folate in wilted vegetables.

ROOT VEGETABLES

Nearly thirty per cent of the average daily intake of vitamin A (in the form of beta-carotene) is provided by vegetables; most of this (18 per cent) by carrots. In contrast, turnips, swedes and parsnips are comparatively good sources of vitamin C, but they contain no beta-carotene.

Effects of cooking

The main purpose of cooking vegetables is to soften the cellular tissue and to gelatinise any starch that may be present so that they can be digested more easily.

Weight changes in preparation and cooking Peeling and trimming may reduce the purchased weight of some vegetables by up to one-third or more (Appendix 3); changes in the weight of most raw vegetables during boiling are small and may be ignored when making calculations from food tables.

Nutrient losses After peeling or shredding, vitamin C is rapidly destroyed by oxidation either directly or by the action of an enzyme present in the plant tissues. This loss can be kept to a minimum by preparing vegetables immediately before use, and by plunging them into boiling water (from which any dissolved oxygen will have been driven off) at the start of the cooking process, when the enzyme will be destroyed.

During cooking, nutrient losses in vegetables (and to a smaller extent in fruit) are mainly caused by the passage of soluble mineral salts and vitamins from the tissues into the cooking water, and by the destruction of some vitamins by heat. Thus, some of the vitamin C and thiamin are inevitably lost when water is used for cooking because they are both heat-sensitive and water-soluble. It is desirable to use small volumes of water for cooking to keep nutrient losses to the minimum. Green vegetables, which have a large surface area, lose on average between 50 and 75 per cent of their vitamin C during cooking. There is a further loss of vitamin C if there is a delay in service and vegetables are kept hot for any length of time. For example, after being kept hot for 30 minutes, cabbage will provide about 60 per cent of its freshly cooked value, and after an hour, only 40 per cent of its original vitamin C. The currently rare practice of adding sodium bicarbonate to the cooking water to maintain a bright green colour in vegetables accelerates losses of vitamin C. Microwaving is a method of cooking vegetables which heats them rapidly using a minimum quantity of water and conserves their texture and colour.

It is not necessary to use salt when boiling vegetables.

Effects of processing

The general effects of processing on the nutritive value of foods are discussed on p. 81.

Freezing does not in itself cause losses of vitamins, but during canning there is some destruction of those vitamins which are unstable to heat (see p. 82).

When sulphite is added to dehydrated vegetables to preserve vitamin C and prevent deterioration of quality during storage, most of the thiamin is destroyed. In general, this loss is not serious because in a mixed diet thiamin is obtained from many other foods.

Fruit

In the diet fruit and fruit juices are nutritionally most important as a major source of vitamin C. These foods together now provide nearly half of all the vitamin C in the British diet. However, the vitamin C content in different fruits varies widely and will always be lower after cooking. Blackcurrants are exceptionally rich, followed by strawberries, kiwis, other soft fruits, oranges, grapefruit and many fruit juices (but not fruit squash unless it is fortified). Many canned fruits, such as pineapples, mandarin oranges and peaches, also supply moderate quantities of vitamin C. Eating apples, bananas, cherries and rhubarb are examples of fruits which contain much less of the vitamin and which do not in this respect compare favourably with green vegetables. Vitamin C may be added to some fruit products such as apple juice and juice drinks. Most fruits also contain sugars and small amounts of beta-carotene, other vitamins and minerals. The sugars in unprocessed fruit are considered to be intrinsic sugars and have not been shown to cause dental caries. However, extrinsic sugars are released from the fruit cells during processing in products such as fruit juices, which can therefore cause dental caries.

Most commercial *fruit juices* are made from concentrated juice and are preserved by UHT treatment (p. 86). There is now also a fairly large production of freshly squeezed juices prepared directly from the fruit, given a mild pasteurisation treatment, and kept chilled before sale. Juice drinks consist of one or more fruit juices, water, sugar and preservatives. Fruit juices and juice drinks retain their vitamin C well during storage, but once the package is opened the vitamin will slowly be lost through oxidation.

Dried fruits such as currants, sultanas, raisins, dates and figs provide energy principally in the form of sugar and are good sources of fibre. They do not contain vitamin C. Prunes and dried apricots are also useful sources of beta-carotene. Dried apricots, figs, prunes, raisins and sultanas are good sources of iron.

Fat spreads and oils

There is now a wide range of margarines, dairy spreads, and reduced- and lower-fat spreads on the market, all of which can be used as butter substitutes. While some margarines consist of a mixture of animal fats and vegetable oils, others contain vegetable oils with a significant proportion of polyunsaturated fatty acids. Almost any edible oil or fat can be used for making fat spreads.

Varying textures can be produced by mixing oils and fats with differing physical properties and by hydrogenation or hardening of oils. Manufacture is by emulsifying the mixture of oils and fats with a salt solution and other constituents such as emulsifiers, flavouring and colouring. *Margarine* by law contains a minimum of 80 per cent fat and not more than 16 per cent water.

Dairy spreads contain variable amounts (but less than 80 per cent) of milk fat such as butter or cream. The fat of *blended spreads* is only part milk fat. *Reduced- or low-fat spreads* generally vary in fat content from about 20 per cent in a very-low-fat spread to about 40 per cent in a low-fat spread and 60 per cent in a reduced-fat spread. However, spreads with only 5 per cent fat are now available; these contain a proportion of a fat replacer (see below).

Vitamins A and D must by law be added to margarine for retail sale. The values required are 800–1000 µg vitamin A (retinol equivalents) and 7.9 µg vitamin D per 100 g. These vitamins are also frequently added to other fat spreads, but this is not obligatory.

Vegetable oils are produced from a variety of plant parts including seeds (e.g. sunflower, rape), grains (e.g. maize or corn), pulses (e.g. soya beans, peanuts), fruits (e.g. olive, palm) and fruit kernels (e.g. olive, palm, coconut). They are traditionally extracted by crushing or milling, but nowadays these processes may be replaced or followed by solvent extraction. Vegetable oils vary in the composition of their fatty acids. They may be sold as a single type, or as a blend of several oils. Some oils, such as sunflower, are high in polyunsaturated fatty acids, while others, such as olive oil, are high in monounsaturated fatty acids.

FAT REPLACERS

Dietary advice to reduce the consumption of fat has stimulated research into ways of reducing the fat content of foods by developing fat replacers which have some of the sensory characteristics of fats, but a lower energy value. Some, including protein-based and carbohydrate-based replacers, are already used in food. A product derived from milk protein (Simplesse), is used in some very-low-fat spreads. Other replacers, including sucrose polyesters, are still awaiting approval for food use.

Sugars and preserves

White sugar provides energy and no other nutrient. Honey and some brown sugars include very small quantities of minerals and certain B-vitamins, but nowhere near enough of the latter to assist with the metabolism of the sugars present (p. 55). Some preserves contain vitamin C, and chocolate contains iron and other nutrients, but the main function of all these foods in the diet is to increase palatability.

Alcohol

The alcohol in alcoholic drinks is rapidly absorbed from the digestive tract and utilised as a source of energy, 1 g of alcohol providing 29 kJ or 7 kcal. Carbohydrate may also be present in varying proportions and this provides additional energy. Consumption of spirits, beer and wine continues to rise and it was reported in 1990 that British adults on an average daily basis obtained 732 kJ (175 kcal) in the case of men, and 200 kJ (48 kcal) in the case of women, from alcoholic drinks. This represented 6.9 and 2.8 per cent, respectively, of their total energy intake. Table 30 gives the energy constituents of some alcoholic drinks.

Chronic alcoholics may obtain a large proportion of their energy intake from alcohol and eat very little food. Beer contains significant amounts of riboflavin and niacin, but spirits contain no vitamins; inevitably the displacement of food by alcohol leads to a marked reduction in the intake of protein, vitamins and many other nutrients.

Table 30. Energy constituents of some alcoholic drinks.

	Average values per 100 ml			
	Alcohol (g)	Carbohydrate (g)	Energy (kJ)	(kcal)
Beer, draught	3.1	2.3	132	32
Lager	3.2	1.5	120	29
Cider, sweet	3.7	4.3	176	42
Sherry, medium	14.8	3.6	489	118
Red wine	9.5	0.3	284	68
White wine, dry	9.1	0.6	275	66
White wine, sweet	10.2	5.9	394	94
Spirits	31.7	0.0	919	222
Liqueurs, medium strength	19.0	32.6	1073	255

1 ml of pure alcohol weighs 0.79 g.

12 Nutritional value of meals and the whole diet

The balanced diet

No single food contains all the essential nutrients the body needs to be healthy and function efficiently. The nutritional value of a person's diet depends on the overall mixture or balance of foods that is eaten over a period of time as well as on the needs of the individual eating them. That is why a balanced diet is one that is likely to include a large number or variety of foods, so adequate intakes of all the nutrients are achieved. Scientists have agreed for many years now that some common health problems, including heart disease and stroke, can be diet-related. Too much saturated fat, for example, is recognised as a contributor to heart disease, and so in this sense a 'balanced' diet also means one with a limited content of fat.

National targets have been set for reductions in the number of people suffering heart disease and stroke and, to help achieve these aims, it will be necessary to reduce fat and saturated fatty acids in the average diet of the population (p.70). Scientific evidence for the relationship between diet and disease is regularly reviewed by expert committees. A person's genes influence their risk of developing diet-related diseases, and other lifestyle factors are also regarded as being very important, particularly exercise and smoking. Diet plays a part in the development or prevention of stroke, since blood pressure is affected by obesity (p. 28) and excessive alcohol intake, and there is some evidence to suggest that in certain people it can also be affected by sodium intake (p. 47). Obese people also have an increased risk of heart disease because they are more likely to have raised levels of blood pressure and blood cholesterol. However, sound nutritional practice can help in preventing these problems by developing eating habits conducive as far as possible to maintaining good health throughout life. For example, when someone is obese through persistent overeating, only a steady reduction in energy intake or increase in energy expenditure, and not sporadic bouts of starvation or exercise, will lead to weight loss that can be maintained. A vitamin deficiency will not result from a diet that is low or lacking in that vitamin for a few days. Nevertheless, the diet is much more likely to contain enough vitamins, especially vitamin C, if fruit, fruit juice or vegetables are eaten every day than if they are eaten only at infrequent intervals. Although heart disease will not result from eating the occasional fat-rich meal, it is wise not to consistently include large amounts of fat, especially saturated fatty acids, in the diet. The maintenance of a sensible and regular eating pattern is important for everyone, so that over the long term a person should ensure that their overall diet is balanced in the way described in this manual, particularly someone whose needs are high or whose appetites may be small, such as a young child, a pregnant woman or an elderly person (see Chapter 13). Food is more likely to be enjoyed, rather than treated simply as something to fill up on in a hurry, if people ensure that their diet is made up of a wide range of different foods so that it is varied and interesting.

Meals and choice of foods

A meal can be arbitrarily defined as the amount of food eaten at one period of time and which provides 850 kJ (200 kcal) or more. This definition covers much more than the popular meaning of the word, which is that of hot, cooked food eaten while sitting down. Different people may eat quite different numbers of meals per day, the arrangements being determined by custom, lifestyle and by working conditions. Many people now do not follow the traditional pattern of three main meals and one or more snacks, but 'graze' or 'snack' at frequent intervals throughout the day. There is evidence that the number of meals taken in a day (and consequently the amount of food eaten at one time) influences the pattern of utilisation of nutrients by the body. However, the balance of nutrients achieved over a period of time is undoubtedly more important in determining a person's nutritional status than the frequency of eating occasions. Nevertheless, it is sensible to try and eat one or more balanced meals each day. Although the amounts of nutrients in different meals may vary, the total intake of each nutrient should meet an individual's needs, ideally each day but certainly over a period of a week, if the food eaten is to be fully satisfactory for health.

Apart from breast milk, which satisfies all a baby's needs for the first few months of life, no single food provides all the nutrients we require. The easiest way of providing an adequate mixture and balance of all the nutrients is to eat a variety of foods chosen from among four main groups: starchy foods, vegetables and fruit, dairy products and meat or alternatives.

People who eat sweets, cakes, biscuits or chocolate between meals or as constant snacks will probably have a reduced appetite for cereals, vegetables or meat at the next meal with the result that they may have a low intake of some nutrients. They may also be more prone to dental decay which can develop from frequent eating of sweet foods. Eating large quantities of high-energy foods at or between meals can result in an undesirable increase in weight if the total daily energy intake exceeds the energy used up and, if these foods are high in saturated fatty acids, may lead to raised blood cholesterol and eventually to the development of heart disease. For adults, the heavy consumption of alcoholic drinks can result in excess energy intake.

BREAKFAST

Because of the length of time since the previous meal, and the consequent low blood sugar level in the morning, it is desirable to eat breakfast before going to school or starting work. It is particularly important for children and people in demanding jobs to have a good breakfast as this helps to keep them alert during the morning. Young children may not be able to satisfy their needs during the rest of the day if breakfast is missed; others may be tempted to fill up on nutrient-poor foods during the morning. Two possible light breakfasts are shown in Table 31. Both are now commonly eaten in Britain, but breakfast 2 provides less fat and saturated fatty acids and much more fibre and vitamin C than breakfast 1. Both provide adequate amounts of energy, protein and a wide variety of vitamins and minerals (not shown). A person who feels unable to eat breakfast immediately on getting up should be encouraged to take a nutritious snack as soon as possible during the morning.

Calculation of nutrients in prepared dishes and meals, using food tables

DISHES

Appendix 3 gives the nutrient composition of many of the ingredients which may be used in mixed dishes. From the recipe, the approximate nutritional value of a dish can then be worked out by arithmetic. To illustrate this, the calculation of the nutritional value of a home-made cheese-and-tomato pizza is shown in Table 32. An allowance has been made for the change in weight and probable loss of thiamin and vitamin C during cooking.

MEALS

It is not uncommon to have a choice between two types of meal: for example, one could be a cooked meal and the other a sandwich-based meal. Many people may now eat the latter at midday rather than the former. Some may not consider that they had eaten a meal at all if the latter is chosen. Table 33 compares the nutrient content of ham sandwiches, a low-fat fruit yogurt and coffee with that of roast chicken, oven chips, peas, canned pineapple and coffee (as calculated from the figures given in Appendix 3). It can be seen that the two meals have a very similar energy value and although the total fat content is higher in the snack meal, saturated fatty acids are at almost the same concentration in both. This particular snack meal has a similar iron content to the cooked meal, but is richer in calcium, vitamin A and thiamin, although it contains less vitamin C and fibre and will contain considerably more sodium unless the cooked meal is salted during cooking or at the table.

Table 31. Comparison of two breakfasts.

	Weight (g)	Energy (kJ)	Energy (kcal)	Protein (g)	Fat (g)	Saturated fatty acids (g)	Fibre (g)	Sodium (mg)	Vitamin C (mg)
Light breakfast 1									
Cornflakes	30	461	108	2.4	0.2	Tr	0.3	333	0.0
Sugar	10	168	39	0.0	0.0	0.0	0.0	0	0.0
Milk, whole	100	275	66	3.2	3.9	2.4	0.0	55	1.0
White bread (1 large thin slice)	31	287	67	2.4	0.4	0.1	0.5	164	0.0
Margarine, polyunsaturated	7	213	52	0.0	5.7	1.1	0.0	56	0.0
Marmalade	15	167	39	0.0	0.0	0.0	0.1	3	1.5
Milk (whole) in 2 cups of tea	50	138	33	1.6	2.0	1.2	0.0	28	0.5
Total		1709	404	9.6	12.2	4.8	0.9	639	3.0
Light breakfast 2									
All Bran	30	333	78	4.2	1.0	0.2	7.3	270	0.0
Sugar	10	168	39	0.0	0.0	0.0	0.0	0	0.0
Milk, semi-skimmed	100	195	46	3.3	1.6	1.0	0.0	55	1.0
Wholemeal bread (thick slice)	44	402	95	4.0	1.1	0.2	2.6	242	0.0
Low fat spread	7	112	27	0.4	2.8	0.8	0.0	46	0.0
Marmalade	15	167	39	0.0	0.0	0.0	0.1	3	1.5
Milk (semi-skimmed) in 2 cups of tea	60	117	28	2.0	1.0	0.6	0.0	33	0.6
Orange juice, small glass	120	184	43	0.6	0.1	0.0	0.1	12	46.8
Total		1678	395	14.5	7.6	2.8	10.1	661	49.9

Table 32. Nutrients in a home-made cheese-and-tomato pizza.

	Weight (g)	Energy (kJ)	Energy (kcal)	Protein (g)	Fat (g)	Saturated fatty acids (g)	Carbo-hydrate (g)
Flour mixture:							
White	75	1087	256	7.1	1.0	0.2	58.3
Wholemeal	75	989	233	9.5	1.7	0.2	47.9
Baking powder	5	35	8	0.3	0.0	0.0	1.9
Margarine, polyunsaturated	50	1519	369	0.1	40.8	8.1	0.5
Milk, semi-skimmed	75	146	35	2.5	1.2	0.8	3.8
Oil, sunflower	10	870	90	0.0	10.0	1.2	0.0
Onions	100	150	36	1.2	0.0	0.0	7.9
Tomatoes, fresh	300	219	51	2.1	0.9	0.3	9.3
Cheddar cheese	150	2562	618	·38.2	51.6	32.6	0.1
Whole pizza, cooked	722	7577	1696	61.0	107.2	43.4	129.7
Per 100g		1049	235	8.4	14.9	6.0	18.0

The pizza weight (722 g) is less than the sum of the ingredients (840 g) owing to the loss of moisture on cooking.

15% of thiamin deducted to allow for loss on cooking; 40% of vitamin C deducted to allow for loss on cooking.

Table 33. Comparison of the nutritional value of a snack and a cooked meal.

	Weight (g)	Energy (kJ)	Energy (kcal)	Protein (g)	Fat (g)	Saturated fatty acids (g)
Snack meal						
Bread, wholemeal (2 slices)	72	658	155	6.6	1.8	0.4
Margarine, polyunsaturated	14	425	103	0.0	11.4	2.3
Ham, canned	70	351	84	12.9	3.6	1.3
Pickle, sweet	20	114	27	0.1	0.1	0.0
Yogurt, low fat, fruit	125	478	113	5.1	0.9	0.5
Coffee, instant	2	8	2	0.3	0.0	0.0
Milk, semi-skimmed	30	59	14	1.0	0.5	0.0
Total		2093	498	26.0	18.3	4.5
Cooked meal						
Roast chicken, meat only	100	621	148	24.8	5.4	1.6
Chips, oven, baked	165	1134	267	5.3	6.9	3.0
Peas, frozen, boiled	70	204	48	4.2	0.6	0.1
Pineapple, canned in juice	80	160	38	0.2	0.0	0.0
Coffee, instant	2	8	2	0.3	0.0	0.0
Milk, semi-skimmed	30	59	14	1.0	0.5	0.0
Total		2186	517	35.8	13.4	4.7

N = not determined.

Fibre (g)	Calcium (mg)	Iron (mg)	Sodium (mg)	Vitamin A (retinol equivalent) (μg)	Thiamin (mg)	Riboflavin (mg)	Niacin equivalent (mg)	Vitamin C (mg)
2.3	105	1.5	2	0	0.23	0.02	2.6	0
6.7	29	2.9	2	0	0.35	0.07	6.1	0
0.0	57	0.0	590	0	0.00	0.00	0.0	0
0.0	2	0.1	400	395	0.00	0.00	0.0	0
0.0	90	0.0	41	17	0.03	0.14	0.7	1
0.0	0	0.0	0	0	0.00	0.00	0.0	0
1.4	25	0.3	3	2	0.13	0.00	1.0	5
3.0	21	1.5	27	320	0.27	0.03	3.3	51
0.0	1080	0.5	1005	544	0.05	0.60	9.1	0
13.4	1409	6.8	2070	1278	0.90	0.86	22.8	34
1.9	195	0.9	287	177	0.13	0.12	3.2	5

Carbohydrate (g)	Fibre (g)	Calcium (mg)	Iron (mg)	Sodium (mg)	Vitamin A (μg)	Thiamin (mg)	Vitamin C (mg)
30.0	4.2	39	1.9	396	0	0.24	0
0.1	0.0	1	0.0	112	126	0.00	0
0.0	0.0	6	0.8	875	0	0.36	0
6.9	0.2	4	0.4	340	8	0.01	0
22.4	N	188	0.1	80	14	0.06	1
0.2	0.0	3	0.1	1	N	0.00	0
1.5	0.0	36	0.0	17	7	0.01	0
61.1	4.4	277	3.3	1821	155	0.68	1
0.0	0.0	9	0.8	81	0	0.08	0
49.2	3.3	20	1.3	87	0	0.18	20
6.8	3.6	25	1.1	1	47	0.18	8
9.8	0.4	6	0.4	1	2	0.07	9
0.2	0.0	3	0.1	1	N	0.00	0
1.5	0.0	36	0.0	17	7	0.01	0
67.5	7.3	99	3.7	188	56	0.52	37

A cold or packed meal is thus not necessarily inferior to a cooked meal; the nutritional values of both depend on the quantity and nutrient content of the items within them.

Allowance for waste

The calculation of the nutritional value of a meal or a diet as actually eaten cannot be made directly from the total amounts of the foods bought from the shops, nor from the total food used in the kitchen. There is always a proportion of waste for which allowance must be made, that is:

1. *Inedible waste*, e.g. egg shells, potato peelings, outer leaves of cabbages, orange peel, bacon rinds, bones and gristle of meat, etc. (See Table 34).

2. *Edible waste*
(a) *Preparation losses*, e.g. batter left in mixing bowls, fat trimmed from meat or left in frying pans, crusts from bread, spilt milk.
(b) *Table waste*, e.g. scraps left on plates.
(c) *Pet food*, e.g. edible scraps fed to domestic pets, garden birds, ducks.
(d) Edible food which has 'gone bad' and is discarded.

INEDIBLE WASTE

Average figures for the inedible waste associated with different foods are given in Appendix 3 as a percentage of the product as listed. For example, 34 per cent of bananas (item 136), as purchased, consists of skin which is not eaten.

The food tables throughout this manual always give the nutrients per 100 g of 'edible portion', and if they are used for calculating the nutritional value of foods where only the purchased weight is known, the percentage of inedible waste must be deducted. For example, the energy value of 1 kg of bananas (purchased weight) will be:

$$10 \times \frac{(100 - 34)}{100} \times (\text{kJ per 100 g from Appendix 3})$$

$$= 10 \times \frac{66}{100} \times 403 = 2660 \text{ kJ} \quad \begin{array}{l}\text{(a similar calculation can be carried out using} \\ \text{kcal per 100 g from Appendix 3)}\end{array}$$

Typical values for the percentage of inedible waste in selected foods are shown in Table 34, but in reality values vary with the exact nature of the food and with its quality. For example, they vary between different cuts and joints of meat and between different sizes and varieties of orange. The values given must therefore be used with discretion.

EDIBLE WASTE

It is often difficult for practical reasons to measure the weight of food actually eaten, for example by a particular individual in a large family or when a meal is

Table 34. Percentage of inedible waste from food as purchased.

Food	%
Bacon, rasher, with rind	6
Chicken, raw, dressed carcase	36
Lamb chop, loin, raw	16
Haddock, steamed with bones and skin	24
Sardines, canned	17
Tuna, canned	19
Eggs, chicken, whole, raw	11
Potatoes, new, raw with skin	11
Potatoes, old, raw with skin	20
Beans, red kidney, canned	36
Beetroot, boiled	20
Cabbage, raw	23
Celery, raw	9
Courgettes, raw	12
Lettuce	26
Mushrooms, raw	3
Onions, raw	9
Peppers, green, raw	16
Processed peas, canned	35
Sweetcorn kernels, canned	18
Watercress	38
Apples, eating	11
Avocado	29
Bananas	34
Blackcurrants, raw	2
Cherries, raw	17
Dates, dried, with stones	16
Grapefruit	32
Grapes	5
Kiwi fruit	14
Mangoes, raw	32
Melon, raw	37
Oranges	30
Peaches, raw	10
Pears, raw	9
Plums, raw	6
Strawberries, raw	5
Almonds, with shells	63

Fresh produce unless specified.

eaten away from home. Estimates of portion sizes and of the loss of edible food may then need to be made before the nutritional adequacy of any diet can be worked out. The average wastage of food in the home in cooking, on plates and from food given to pets has been found to be between 5 and 10 per cent, but of course the amount varies from food to food and from family to family. Wastage can also be high in some catering establishments.

Planning balanced meals and nutritionally adequate diets

The provision of palatable and acceptable meals must be the first consideration; only within this framework can planning for good nutrition be effective.

A balanced meal is one which provides adequate amounts of protein and of all the minerals and vitamins as well as energy. It should also provide fibre, and should be limited in its fat, sugar and salt contents. At least one balanced meal should be eaten every day.

The main sources of each nutrient are discussed in Chapters 2, 3, 4, 7 and 8, and the detailed composition of a range of foods is given in Appendix 3. Most foods contain a wide variety of nutrients, and most minerals and vitamins are present in a wide variety of common foods. Thus the simplest way to meet nutritional standards is to eat a varied diet containing a wide selection of different types of food.

Experience and custom have influenced food choice in such a way that traditional meals are generally nutritionally satisfactory as well as good to eat; nevertheless to be sure that this is maintained, now that we rely to a greater extent on snacks and convenience foods, certain rules can be followed. To help make this easier, the Government has produced a set of eight guidelines for a healthy diet and a National Food Guide (see Appendix 6). In general:

(a) Starchy foods, such as cereals, potatoes, yams, rice and pasta which provide energy, fibre, vitamins and minerals, should form the main part of most meals and snacks.

(b) The starchy basis of a meal should be accompanied by selections from foods such as meat, fish, eggs, pulses, nuts, milk and dairy products, rich in protein, vitamins and minerals.

(c) The daily diet should contain plenty of fruit and vegetables, which are good sources of some vitamins and minerals not commonly found in other foods, and of fibre.

(d) Foods rich in energy, such as butter, margarine, lower-fat spreads, cream, fried foods, jam, cakes, pastries, biscuits and other foods rich in fat and sugar, and alcoholic drinks, should be eaten only in limited amounts which will satisfy appetite and maintain correct body weight.

The Reference Nutrient Intakes of selected major nutrients for groups of people of different ages are given on p. 69, and these figures may be used as a guide when planning diets. The Estimated Average Requirements for fat and

110

carbohydrate for adults are summarised in Table 26 on p. 70. As a rule of thumb, on average, fat should not provide more than 35 per cent of dietary energy for adults, nor saturated fatty acids more than 10 per cent of dietary energy. By implication, the total carbohydrate in the diet should provide about 50 per cent of the food energy, with no more than about 10 per cent coming from non-milk extrinsic sugars. Children under five years of age who are not able to eat large quantities of bulky foods, may not obtain sufficient energy unless they are given energy-dense foods. It is therefore not wise to limit their fat intake too much (note that human breast milk derives 54 per cent of its energy from fat and 26 per cent from saturated fatty acids).

The adult diet should provide 18 g per day of fibre as non-starch polysaccharides. Wholemeal versions of cereals provide more fibre than refined products. The sodium intake of adults should be on average about 2.3 g per day (equivalent to about 6 g per day of salt) and this can be achieved from the salt already present in food. Most people should try to eat fewer salty foods and use less salt in cooking and at the table.

In practice it will be found that certain meals such as the traditional Sunday lunch are likely to be rich in fat and other nutrients whereas others, including breakfasts for many people, will provide a counterbalance. It is the total nutrient intake over at least one day (as in the example given on page 124), and preferably a week, that should be assessed; and even then it is the balance of the diet in the longer term which is really important for health.

Planning meals in relation to cost

Within this general framework it is usually necessary to consider the relative cost of different sources of nutrients. Allowance must also be made for the effects of cooking on nutritive value.

Great savings in the cost of eating can be made with a thorough knowledge of food composition and nutritional value for money. For example, cheaper cuts of lean meat have practically the same nutritional value as the more expensive cuts although they may take longer to cook. Many meat products also provide good nutritional value for money. However, fatty meat and some meat products may prove relatively expensive if large quantities of fat have to be trimmed off before cooking or discarded after cooking. Again, cheaper fatty fish such as mackerel have a similar nutritional value to a more expensive fatty fish such as salmon. The cheaper fresh vegetables such as cabbage, carrots and potatoes are often much better value for money than many canned or frozen vegetables. Fresh citrus fruits are very convenient sources of vitamin C and are also fairly cheap. Cheese, eggs or pulses can take the place of meat in a main course.

Section 3 of Appendix 4 shows how a comparison can be made between the amounts of protein, vitamins or other nutrients bought for one monetary unit

Table 35. Cheap sources of energy and nutrients (in approximate[a] order, with the cheapest first).

Energy	Vegetable oil, sugar, margarine, oatmeal, butter, white bread, dried pulses, wholemeal bread, brown bread, rice, pasta, potatoes, biscuits, nuts, breakfast cereals.
Protein	Pulses, white bread, wholemeal bread, brown bread, liver, pasta, canned beans, eggs, herring fillets, uncooked chicken, milk, minced beef, cheese, potatoes, frozen peas, rice.
Carbohydrate	Sugar, white bread, oatmeal, rice, potatoes, brown bread, wholemeal bread, pasta, pulses, biscuits, breakfast cereals, dried fruit, canned beans, soft drinks.
Vitamin C	Frozen fruit and fruit products, instant potato (many are fortified with vitamin C), oranges, fruit juices, fresh soft fruit, other citrus fruits, canned tomatoes, turnips, swedes, fresh potatoes, tomatoes, frozen peas, fresh green vegetables.
Vitamin D	Margarine, reduced-fat spread, canned salmon, canned tuna, fatty fish, milk (instant dried skimmed milk), eggs, fortified breakfast cereals, butter, liver.
Fibre	Dried pulses, wholemeal bread, high-fibre breakfast cereals, canned beans, frozen peas, fresh rhubarb, muesli, brown bread, potatoes, white bread, fresh pears, nuts and nut products, fresh apples, fresh green vegetables.
Riboflavin	Liver, breakfast cereals, milk, eggs, paté, yogurt, brown bread, wholemeal bread, cheese, potatoes.
Niacin equivalent	Liver, dried pulses, meat and yeast extracts, canned tuna, fortified breakfast cereals, nuts and nut products, white bread, corned beef, uncooked chicken, brown bread, potatoes, minced beef, frozen peas, wholemeal bread, sausages.
Calcium	Milk, white bread, cheese, brown bread, wholemeal bread, ice cream, eggs.
Iron	Dried pulses, liver, oatmeal, fortified breakfast cereals, bread (wholemeal, brown, white), canned/frozen peas, potatoes, eggs, biscuits.
Thiamin	Oatmeal, potatoes, fortified breakfast cereals, dried pulses, bread (wholemeal, brown, white), frozen peas, liver, oranges, pork, bacon/ham.

[a] As at 1992. When harvests are badly affected by weather conditions, the nutritional value-for-money provided by some of these foods may decline.

(in this case a penny) for any food by using the food composition tables and the price of the food. The precise relationship between foods will vary according to the time of year and current prices, but Table 35 gives a general idea of some cheap sources of certain nutrients. It is important to realise that a cheap source of one nutrient may not be a cheap food in the context of the whole diet, as with sugar where only one nutrient is supplied. Bread, pasta, rice, breakfast cereals, milk, cheese, offals, potatoes, peas and beans, on the other hand, all supply several nutrients cheaply and are thus very good value for money.

Planning meals for the week ahead is most important in food budgeting. Careful shopping, correct preparation and storage of food, and a knowledge of basic cookery skills all play a part in using the available money to the best advantage.

13   Needs of particular groups of people

Infants and young children

Infants are unique in that they must rely on a single food, milk, to satisfy all their nutritional needs. Breast milk is ideal for several reasons:

(a) All the nutrients are present in the right amount for human infants, and in a readily absorbed form. Those nutrients which are low, such as iron and copper, are those which are already stored in large amounts in the infant's liver.

(b) It contains several natural agents which protect against disease.

(c) It is clean, cannot be prepared incorrectly, and does not cause allergies.

A mother should therefore try to breastfeed her baby for at least two weeks, and ideally for 4–6 months. Few mothers are unable to breastfeed. Those who cannot do so for medical reasons or who prefer not to can use formulas, usually based on cow's milk, which have been modified so that they are more like human milk. Since the immature kidneys of young infants are unable to adapt to high concentrations of protein and some minerals it is very important to make up these feeds exactly according to the instructions so that they are not too concentrated. In hot weather extra drinks of water may be needed but sugary drinks and juices can harm the developing teeth.

Solid foods should not be introduced before 4 months of age. There is no advantage to the baby to do so and there may be some risks of developing allergies and of becoming obese. From about 6 months onwards the mother may gradually introduce infant cereal foods, puréed fruit and vegetables, egg yolk, and even finely divided meat (using no added salt or sugar). By about 12–18 months, the infant can eat a mixed diet not very different from that of the rest of the family. Whole milk will continue to be very important until the age of 2, after which semi-skimmed milk may be introduced but less will be drunk as more solid foods are eaten. Skimmed milk is not suitable for children under 5.

Studies have shown that a significant proportion of infants and young children between 9 months and $3\frac{1}{2}$ years of age have low iron intakes (below the Lower Reference Nutrient Intake). Although it has not yet been established whether children with habitually low intakes are deficient in iron, it is wise to include rich sources of iron among the foods provided for this age group. Some good sources of iron are listed in Part 1.

Drops containing vitamins A, C and D may also be useful (and are provided free for those in need) as may fluoride supplements in areas where the drinking water is low in fluoride.

Schoolchildren

Schoolchildren are growing fast and are also very active. Tables 24 and 25 give the Estimated Average Requirements (EAR) for energy, and Reference Nutrient Intakes (RNI) for major nutrients for groups of children of different ages, and show that these are high in relation to their body size compared with those of adults. For example, the EAR for 7- to 10-year-old girls for energy and their RNI for thiamin are nearly as high as those for grown women in most occupations. The big appetites of some children usually reflect a real nutritional need rather than greed. Because of their smaller size compared with adults, and correspondingly smaller stomachs, it is important that children should eat meals which are not too bulky. Bread, milk, cheese, meat, fish, liver, eggs, fruit, green vegetables and potatoes are all excellent sources of a number of nutrients. Milk, whether whole, semi-skimmed or skimmed, is one of the best sources of calcium, riboflavin and protein. Children should be taught sensible eating habits from an early age: biscuits, sweets, soft drinks, chips and crisps should not displace other more useful foods too often, either at home or at school. Sweet and sticky foods and snacks eaten frequently between meals are one cause of the dental decay found in many British schoolchildren. Children should be encouraged to clean their teeth every day with a fluoride toothpaste.

Adolescents

The nutrient needs of adolescents are higher in many respects than those of any other group. Healthy adolescents have large appetites and it is important that they should satisfy them with food of high nutritional value in the form of well-balanced meals (p. 110) rather than by too many snacks rich in fat, sugar or salt. Obesity among schoolchildren is common and this may continue into adult life. It is more sensible to prevent obesity than try to correct it by periodically eating little or no food; excessive dieting can be dangerous (p. 30). There is also evidence that adolescent obesity is partly due to a general decrease in physical activity and hence in energy expenditure rather than to an excessive energy intake. A knowledge of nutrition and the incentive to apply this knowledge in practice is likely to benefit the health of young people for the rest of their lives.

Adolescent girls who become pregnant are at particular risk of developing nutrient deficiencies, needing additional nutrients for their baby's growth as well as for their own.

Adults

Many adults in Britain are more likely to be at risk of overnutrition than of undernutrition. Those adults who wish to reduce their intakes of energy or of fat and saturated fatty acids to reduce their risk of premature heart disease will find information throughout this manual which will help them to achieve this. Anyone needing to make changes to their diet will find these easier to follow if they are shared with other members of the family or with friends. There is also information for those who wish to reduce their intakes of sugars and salt and to increase their intake of fibre.

In general, healthy, well-balanced diets are high in starchy foods and fruit and vegetables, contain moderate amounts of meat or its alternatives and milk and dairy foods and only small quantities of foods with high concentrations of fat and sugar. The carbohydrate from cereal products including bread, rice and pasta, and from potatoes or other tubers such as yams, is needed to make good the energy lost from any reduction in fats and sugars. These foods will also contribute fibre, but may add to the total salt intake unless less salt is used on the plate and in their preparation as well as in that of vegetables and meat dishes. It is always wise to evaluate the whole diet before making any changes so that the intake of other nutrients, as well as the nutrient of concern, and the foods which chiefly contribute to these intakes, are known. There would be little point, for example, in reducing an individual's fat intake further if their diet is already low in fat, or of reducing their intake of a favourite food if this contributes little to their overall fat intake. COMA has recommended that reducing fat intakes should not result in higher intakes of foods rich in sugars or salt.

It is also important to keep alcohol intake under control. Regular consumption of between 3 and 4 units a day or less for men and 2 and 3 units a day or less for women will not significantly increase the risk to a person's health over time. Drinking more than this on a regular basis over time, however, brings increasing risks to health. Women who are, or are trying to become, pregnant should not drink more than 1 or 2 units of alcohol once or twice a week. Light drinking of between 1 and 2 units a day, however, can exert a beneficial protective effect against coronary heart disease for people at risk, namely men over forty and women who have gone through the menopause. A unit of alcohol is half a pint of beer, a small glass of sherry, a glass of wine or a single measure of spirits.

Pregnancy and lactation

A woman's nutritional needs increase during pregnancy and lactation (p. 27). This is not only because her diet must provide for the growth and development of her child, but also because other physiological changes occur to ensure that sufficient nutrients are available for the child (such as the laying down of new tissues in the woman's own body) and that the mother has enough energy to carry the extra weight. Much of the weight gain during the early part of pregnancy is due to the accumulation of fat which provides an energy store to meet the additional demands of the growing foetus and the breastfed infant.

Approximate weight of a foetus and infant at various ages

Conception	0	kg
4½ months pregnancy	0.5	kg
9 months pregnancy (birth)	3.5	kg
4½ months after birth	7	kg

It is most important that the mother's diet contains sufficient energy, protein, iron, calcium, folate and vitamins C and D (and liquid during lactation) for building the baby's muscular tissues, bones and teeth, and for the formation of haemoglobin; if it does not, her own stores of nutrients may be reduced. Some good sources of these nutrients are given in Part 1. In practice most of these extra nutrients will be obtained simply by satisfying the appetite with a good mixed diet including plenty of bread, fruit and vegetables, dairy products and meat or its alternatives. Extra folic acid/folate before and during pregnancy is needed by some women to decrease the risk of occurrence of neural tube defects in their babies. As it is not known who is at risk, in the case of first-time pregnancies or those with normal children, all women planning a pregnancy are advised to take a daily supplement of 0.4 mg of folic acid before becoming pregnant as well as eating folate-rich foods. Those who have already had an affected child should take 4 or 5 mg folic acid each day (see p. 60). Special supplements of iron may also be recommended during pregnancy and drops containing vitamins A, C and D are available to those in need. However, pregnant women are advised not to take supplements containing vitamin A or eat foods such as liver that may be extremely rich in vitamin A, except on the advice of their doctor, due to the possible risk of birth defects (see p. 53). A good knowledge of nutrition is invaluable during pregnancy and lactation and will also help the mother to teach sound eating habits to her child in due course.

Older people

There is very little difference between the nutritional requirements of most older people and the younger adult. However, as age progresses and body weight and energy expenditure decrease, people tend to eat less and hence may find it difficult to satisfy all the nutrient requirements. It is important, therefore, that older people are encouraged to maintain a good energy intake unless they are obese. They should also have foods which are concentrated sources of protein, vitamins and minerals. The EARs for energy for populations of people aged 60 or over are shown in Table 24. A healthy weight can be more readily maintained and recovery from illness or injury will be more rapid if older people are also encouraged to take plenty of gentle exercise. In 1992 the Committee on Medical Aspects of Food Policy (COMA) recommended that older people should adopt diets that will help to moderate their blood cholesterol levels to reduce their risk of heart disease. As with younger adults, therefore, older people should not eat too much fat or saturated fatty acids and they should aim to eat meals based on starchy foods. Encouraging them to include oily fish in their diets would help to reduce their risk of thrombosis (development of a blood clot which may block narrowed arteries and result in a heart attack). COMA has also recommended that, on average, older people should follow the DRV for non-milk extrinsic sugars which would help them to retain their own teeth (for those without dentures or with only partial dentures), consume a more varied diet than would be possible with high sugar intakes, and prevent possible disorders of their metabolism arising from a high sucrose load. However, when very elderly people are unwell, sugar in amounts additional to recommendations may help to make their food more palatable and encourage them to eat. Older people would also benefit from eating plenty of fruit and vegetables, items that are often lacking in their diets, in order to prevent vitamin C deficiency. Foods rich in fibre can also help to prevent constipation.

Those who live alone should be encouraged to prepare at least one meal a day of good nutritional quality, stressing that this does not necessarily have to be a hot meal, and to supplement this with foods such as milk, cheese, yogurt, eggs, breakfast cereals, bread, and fruits or fruit juices rich in vitamin C which need little preparation. It is a good idea, for those times when an elderly person is unwell or when the weather is bad and they are unable to shop, to have a store cupboard of essential items such as powdered or UHT milk, breakfast cereals, cans of fish such as sardines, canned fruit, vegetables, pulses and milk puddings, UHT fruit juices and dried fruit. Items such as frozen ready meals and a supply of bread and vegetables can be kept in where a freezer is available. Whenever possible, older people should go outside for a short time in the summer months and expose their forearms, hands and face to the sun. For those who do not have the benefit of sunlight because they are completely housebound or do not wish to remove enveloping clothes, a good dietary source of vitamin D such as margarine, eggs or fatty fish (e.g. sardines, mackerel) is important, and they should seek advice from their doctor about the need for an additional supplement of vitamin D.

Slimmers

Energy needs and food consumption have been discussed in Chapter 5.

Planning a slimming diet is a matter of individual preference. Essentially, the energy intake needs to be cut down by 2–4 MJ (500–1000 kcal) each day to achieve a weekly weight loss of 0.5–1.0 kg (1–2 lb). Other nutrients should still reach recommended levels. It is often convenient to cut out fatty and sugary foods such as cakes, sweets, preserves, biscuits and some puddings as well as alcohol, as these tend to be sources of energy rather than nutrients. Low- or reduced-fat and sugar products, now readily available, can be substituted for traditionally high-fat and sugar foods. Fat can be trimmed from meat, and foods can be boiled or grilled and not fried. Foods high in water or fibre can induce feelings of fullness and so help to reduce the desire for more food.

Effective slimming diets are all basically low energy or 'low calorie' diets, though they vary in how this is achieved. A good plan is to base meals on a modest helping of lean meat, fish, eggs or reduced-fat cheese with liberal amounts of fruits and vegetables and moderate amounts of bread, potatoes, rice and pasta. Eating three or four meals a day gives better results than eating the same amount of food at one or two meals only. Including breakfast, ideally based on a whole-grain breakfast cereal with skimmed milk or yogurt and fruit, helps to avoid mid-morning hunger. As it may take several months to reach the desired healthy weight, a slimming diet should be sensible and palatable enough to be tolerated for this length of time. After this, it is advisable to keep to the changes made to the diet whilst slimming and gradually increase the energy content until the new healthy weight is maintained. Cranky diets based on only one or two foods may be successful in the short term but are hard to adhere to as they are unrealistic, dull, and do not teach healthy eating habits; they can also be deficient in a range of nutrients and therefore dangerous. Very-low-calorie diets (VLCDs) (less than 3.4 MJ (800 kcal) per day) are unsuitable for infants, children, adolescents, pregnant or lactating women, the elderly and people with certain medical conditions, e.g. heart disease.

There are times when it is difficult to reduce food intake especially on social occasions but by planning to eat less for a day or two beforehand, it is possible to enjoy food on such occasions without weight gain. Keeping to a slimming diet can sometimes be made easier by joining a slimmers' group, and weight loss is improved by being physically active.

Vegetarians

Vegetarians do not eat meat and most do not eat fish, but the majority consume some animal products – the most important of which are milk, cheese and eggs. Such diets may be rather bulky and lower in energy than a mixed diet because most vegetables have a high water content but, in general, their nutritional values are very similar to those of mixed diets.

A much smaller group, *vegans*, eat no foods of animal origin at all. Human nutrient requirements, with the exception of vitamin B_{12} (p. 58), can be met by a diet composed entirely of plant foods, but to do so it must be carefully planned using a wide selection of foods. A mixture of plant proteins derived from cereals, peas, beans and nuts will provide enough protein of good quality, but special care is needed to ensure that sufficient energy, calcium, iron, riboflavin, vitamin B_{12} and vitamin D are also available. Yeast extract is a good source of some of the B-vitamins including vitamin B_{12} which are otherwise found mainly in foods of animal origin. In extreme cases, such as Zen macrobiotic diets where little but whole-grain cereals are eaten, intakes of calcium, iron, vitamin B_{12} and vitamin C are likely to be too low for health.

Some people, both vegetarian and non-vegetarian, prefer to eat only or mainly 'organic' foods. All foods, being derived from plants or animals, are organic; and all foods because they provide nutrients, are conducive to health when eaten as part of a balanced diet as described in this manual. The word 'organic' has, however, come to acquire the restricted meaning of foods grown without the use of inorganic fertilisers, pesticides or herbicides, and either not processed or processed without the use of additives. The use of these substances aids the production and economic distribution of the food needed for our dense urban population and is controlled by legislation (p. 153). There is little difference between organic and non-organic produce in terms of nutritional value which is largely determined by the species of plant or animal.

Ethnic groups

In general the traditional diets of ethnic communities provide adequate nourishment to those who consume them. Recent immigrants to the UK, who have difficulty adapting their traditional diets and customs (see Table 36) to local circumstances, may have special dietary problems. In particular, Asian vegetarian groups may have very low intakes of vitamin D. As exposure to sunlight (especially by women and children) may also be low due to customs of dress and because they tend to remain indoors, rickets and osteomalacia sometimes develop. Good sources of vitamin D should therefore be included in sufficient quantity in the diet and vitamin supplements may be necessary. Iron deficiency anaemia sometimes occurs among women and children, particularly in the Asian community, since the iron content of certain traditional diets may also be low.

Diabetics

Diabetes is a metabolic disorder which reduces the ability of the body to control the amount of glucose in the blood (p. 39). It is important for diabetics to avoid the large rises in blood glucose which can result from eating readily absorbed carbohydrate but this requires control rather than a reduction in total carbohydrate intake. Indeed, many Asian diabetics live well with 60 per cent or more of their diet as carbohydrate from rice or chapatis,

Table 36. Dietary restrictions practised by religious and ethnic groups.

Hindus	No beef	Mostly vegetarian; fish rarely eaten; no alcohol	Period of fasting common
Muslim	No pork	Meat must be 'Halal'; no shellfish eaten; no alcohol	Regular fasting, including Ramadan for one month
Sikhs	No beef	Meat must be killed by 'one blow to the head'; no alcohol	Generally less rigid eating restrictions than Hindus and Muslims
Jews	No pork	Meat must be kosher; only fish with scales and fins eaten	Meat and dairy foods must not be consumed together
Rastafarians	No animal products except milk may be consumed	Foods must be 'I-tal' or alive, so no canned or processed foods eaten; no salt added; no coffee or alcohol	Food should be organic

Halal meat is dedicated to God by a Muslim present at the killing. Kosher meat must be slaughtered by a Rabbinical-licensed person and then soaked and salted.

whereas traditional low-carbohydrate diets, being high in fat, may have contributed to the prevalence of heart disease in British diabetics. It is particularly important for diabetics to control their weight since obesity reduces the body's ability to metabolise glucose and can therefore worsen diabetic control. Otherwise they should eat diets similar to those recommended for other adults.

Other special diets

The principles set out in this manual hold in general for all healthy individuals. There are, however, a few people who possess personal idiosyncrasies causing reactions to certain foods, for example, eggs, shellfish or strawberries. In some cases, such as allergy to nuts, inadvertent consumption can result in the rapid onset of anaphylactic shock which, unless treated immediately, can be fatal. In conditions such as coeliac disease (pp. 22, 37) or lactose intolerance (p. 11), a special diet should be followed and, when certain drugs are taken, the avoidance of specific foods (e.g. cheese) is necessary. These allergies and illnesses are a medical rather than a nutritional problem.

Summary: assessing the adequacy of a diet

It is important not only that all the essential nutrients should be present in the foods eaten, but also that they should be present in the amounts required by different people. To find out whether a particular diet is nutritionally adequate, three things must be known:

(a) What foods were eaten?

(b) How much of each food was eaten?

(c) What kind of person or people ate the foods? Were they men, women, adolescents or children, and were they very active or sedentary? Were any of the women pregnant or nursing a baby?

When the answers to these questions are known, daily nutrient intakes can then be compared with the Dietary Reference Values and any other appropriate guidelines. It must, however, be emphasised that the RNIs for minerals and vitamins are high enough to cover the needs of practically all healthy people; someone who obtains less than the RNI is not necessarily deficient in that nutrient. An individual will only give cause for concern if they are consistently obtaining less than the LRNI.

Four important methods of measuring food consumption are:

(a) Measuring the amount of food and drink purchased both for the home and from catering establishments by, for example, a family during one week. When the amount of food bought is recorded, as in the National Food Survey, it is important to follow up by finding out how much of it is eaten, how much goes into or out of the store cupboard or freezer, how many people ate it, and how much is wasted in preparing meals and on the plate.

(b) Recalling, preferably with expert help, all the foods eaten in the previous 24 hours or 3 days. This is the least time-consuming method, but it is easy to forget important foods and hard to estimate quantities accurately. It may be supplemented, or replaced, with a diet history which records a person's recollection of their 'typical' 7-day eating pattern.

(c) Weighing all the foods eaten or drunk over a long enough period (usually a whole week). Provided that the diet is not changed to accommodate the complex recording procedure, this should be the most precise method of assessing the value of anyone's diet. However, some people may, consciously or otherwise, make alterations to their normal diet during the survey week.

(d) Responding to a food frequency questionnaire to say how often each food from a list is eaten in terms of x times per day/per week/per month. It may also include assessment of the quantity of food consumed on each eating occasion. Foods may be singled out for study if it is not necessary to assess the total diet and it is quick and easy to complete. However, it is not accurate, especially for the quantities consumed.

It is easy to determine the weights of standard or pre-packaged items, and for meals served in some canteens or restaurants it may be possible to weigh all the components of duplicates of the meal. More care is needed to evaluate variable items such as stews in either the domestic or catering contexts. It is also important to remember that the nutrient content of foods may vary from the average values shown in this manual.

As an example of the way in which a diet can be evaluated, the daily pattern of snacks and meals which might have been eaten by a young man in a sedentary occupation has been set out in a systematic way in Table 37. The nutrients provided by these quantities of each of these foods must be calculated using food tables such as that in Appendix 3. The results can be summarised meal by meal as in Table 38, or the contribution of each food to each nutrient can be listed if the evaluation covers only a short period.

Table 37. Menu for one day for a young sedentary man.

	Weight (g)		Weight (g)
Breakfast		*Evening meal*	
Orange juice	120	Spaghetti	220
Cornflakes	50	Bolognese sauce	250
Milk, semi-skimmed	146	Cheddar cheese	10
Sugar with cornflakes	10	Lettuce	30
Brown bread	46	Tomato	65
Margarine, polyunsaturated	14	Ice cream	60
Marmalade	30	Peaches, canned in syrup	120
1 cup of tea			
Milk, semi-skimmed with tea	30		
Sugar with tea	4		
Lunch (sandwiches)		*Snacks throughout the day*	
Soft grain bread	72	2 cups of coffee	
Margarine	14	Milk, semi-skimmed with coffee	60
Tuna, canned in brine	45	Sugar with coffee	10
Mayonnaise	15	1 packet crisps	28
Banana	100	1 apple	112
1 can of carbonated drink	337	2 digestive biscuits	26
		1 pint lager	574

The intakes of nutrients can then be compared with the Dietary Reference Values for such a person, and with an understanding of the principles set out in this manual the significance of any departures from these values can be assessed. In the instance given in Table 37:

Calcium, iron, thiamin and vitamin C intakes are well above the RNIs for these nutrients. In general it is easier for men to achieve these levels than women because they eat larger quantities of food. The *sodium* content of the day's meals is more than twice the suggested RNI for an adult and is much higher than the COMA recommended average adult intake of 2.3 g per day. It could be advisable for this young man to moderate his sodium intake by, for

Table 38. Nutrient content of a menu for a young sedentary man.

	Energy (kJ)	Energy (kcal)	Protein (g)	Fat (g)	Saturated fat (g)	Carbo-hydrate (g)	Fibre (g)	Calcium (mg)	Iron (mg)	Sodium (mg)	Thiamin (mg)	Vitamin C (mg)
Breakfast	2716	641	14.3	15.6	4.3	118.4	2.4	288.0	4.9	1030	0.79	52
Lunch	2715	644	17.5	24.4	4.4	94.7	3.3	132.8	2.5	676	0.19	11
Evening meal	3441	821	33.7	38.3	12.9	91.3	7.1	233.5	5.5	1199	0.33	29
Snacks	2348	561	6.8	17.0	5.4	67.0	4.0	133.9	1.5	515	0.12	15
Total	11220	2667	72.3 / 10.8[a]	95.3 / 32.2[a]	27.0 / 9.1[a]	371.4 / 52.2[a]	16.8	788.2	14.4	3420	1.43	107
EAR (DH 1991)	10600	2550	44.4	33.0[a]	10.0[a]	47.0[a]	18.0	525.0	6.7		0.75	25
RNI (DH 1991)			55.5					700.0	8.7	1600	1.00	40
LRNI (DH 1991)								400.0	4.7	575	0.60	10

[a] As a percentage of total energy.
See also Table 33.

example, substituting a lower-sodium cereal for cornflakes, replacing a salty snack like crisps with a low-fat yogurt or fruit, and adding less salt to the main dish during cooking.

The *energy* intake is quite close to the EAR for a man aged between 19 and 40 with a physical activity level of 1.4. However, many sedentary men have lower energy intakes than this, and it is possible that he may gain weight if such a meal pattern were eaten regularly. The proportion of total energy derived from *protein* is 10.8 per cent which is acceptable. The proportion of the total energy intake derived from *fat* is 32.2 per cent, from *saturated fat* 9.1 per cent and from *carbohydrate* 52.2 per cent. If the total fat and saturated fatty acid intakes were maintained at or about this level over the course of time, the fat content of the whole diet would be very satisfactory. Hence if he wished to treat himself to a chocolate bar on another day he might want to substitute low-fat yogurt for ice cream in the evening and fresh fruit or salad items for the crisps or biscuits during snack times. An increase in his intake of starch-rich foods at the expense of sugar could improve his intake of *fibre as NSP* (which is a little low), especially if whole-grain products are consumed. Alternatively, it could be raised by, for example, substituting a high-fibre cereal for cornflakes at breakfast.

It should be recalled that the DRVs for fat, saturated fatty acids and carbohydrate are meant to be applied to populations of people rather than individuals. Therefore it is desirable for a group of men of this age and lifestyle who, as individuals, vary in their nutrient needs, to consume on average over time a diet which achieves the DRVs, rather than each individual aiming to achieve the DRVs every day. Nevertheless, if each individual tries to make changes towards a more healthy diet, the more likelihood there is that the population as a whole will achieve the DRVs.[1]

---

[1] To help people to attain a sensible balance and variety of foods for a healthy diet, the UK Government has apportioned foods into five groups, namely bread, other cereals and potatoes, fruit and vegetables, meat, fish and alternatives, milk and dairy foods, and fatty and sugary foods. A National Food Guide has been designed in the form of a plate divided into segments representing these groups in the proportions in which they should be eaten over the course of about a week to achieve the DRVs. The National Food Guide is represented in Appendix 6.

APPENDICES

Appendix 1 Common measures and conversion factors

Although the labels of most pre-packed foods give their weight in grams, many fresh foods are weighed in imperial units and many individuals still use pounds (weight), pints, inches, etc. Furthermore energy has long been measured in calories, but the SI units joules are also being used. The conversion factors below show the relationships between these units.

WEIGHT

1 milligram (mg)	= 1000 micrograms (µg)	
1 gram (g)	= 1000 mg	= 0.035 oz
1 kilogram (kg)	= 1000 g	= 2.20 lb
1 ounce (oz)	= 28.35 g	
1 pound (lb)	= 453.6 g	

VOLUME

| 1 litre | = 1000 millilitres (ml) | = 1.76 pt |
| 1 pint (pt) | = 20 fluid oz | = 568 ml |

LENGTH

1 metre (m)	= 100 centimetres (cm)	= 1000 millimetres (mm)
		= 39.4 in
1 inch (in)	= 2.54 cm	
1 foot (ft)	= 0.3048 m	

ENERGY

1 kilojoule (kJ)	= 1000 joules (J)	
1 megajoule (MJ)	= 1000 kJ	= 239 kcal
1 kilocalorie (kcal)	= 4.184 kJ	

Appendix 2 Equations for estimating the basal metabolic rate (BMR)

BMR (MJ/day)

Males	10–17 years	$BMR = 0.074W + 2.754$
	18–29 years	$BMR = 0.063W + 2.896$
	30–59 years	$BMR = 0.048W + 3.653$
	Over 60 years	$BMR = 0.049W + 2.459$
Females	10–17 years	$BMR = 0.056W + 2.898$
	18–29 years	$BMR = 0.062W + 2.036$
	30–59 years	$BMR = 0.034W + 3.538$
	Over 60 years	$BMR = 0.038W + 2.755$

BMR (kcal/day)

Males	10–17 years	$BMR = 17.7W + 657$
	18–29 years	$BMR = 15.1W + 692$
	30–59 years	$BMR = 11.5W + 873$
Females	10–17 years	$BMR = 13.4W + 692$
	18–29 years	$BMR = 14.8W + 487$
	30–59 years	$BMR = 8.3W + 846$

W = body weight (kg)

Example: A woman, 40 years old, who weighs 62kg

$$BMR = (0.034 \times 62) + 3.538$$
$$= 2.108 + 3.538 = 5.646$$
$$= 5.7 \text{ MJ/day}$$

or $$BMR = (8.3 \times 62) + 846 = 515 + 846$$
$$= 1361 \text{ kcal/day}$$

Appendix 3   Composition of food

Typical values for the amounts of a number of nutrients in a wide variety of raw and cooked foods are shown in the following table. Each value is the amount per 100 g of the edible part of the food as described. The information is based on the fifth revised edition of *McCance and Widdowson's The Composition of Foods* (1991), which gives details of more foods and more nutrients than are shown here. Individual samples of food can differ considerably depending on the season of the year; therefore, any information given on the label by the manufacturers should be more appropriate for that particular product than the more general values in this Appendix.

Allowance may need to be made for wastage in foods that are weighed raw. The values given here predict the proportion of each food as listed that cannot be eaten. Thus for raw chicken it is the amount of bone and skin likely to be in the whole or joint of a chicken to be cooked, but for slices of roast chicken there would be no wastage. Some individuals may, however, choose not to eat some of the fat or to discard any parts of a fruit that are bruised, and an additional allowance may have to be made for this.

The energy value of each food is given in kilojoules (kJ) and kilocalories (kcal), and both have been calculated from the protein, fat and carbohydrate content as on p. 30. The figures for vitamin A are given in the form of retinol equivalents (p. 53). They are thus expressed in the same form as in the *Dietary Reference Values for Food Energy and Nutrients for the United Kingdom* (1991). Available carbohydrate is given as its monosaccharide equivalent (p. 9). Appendix 4 provides examples of the use of this table.

Table 3.1. Composition per 100 g of edible portion.

No.	Food	Inedible waste (%)	Water (g)	Energy (kJ)	Energy (kcal)	Protein (g)	Fat (g)	Saturated fatty acids (g)
	Cereals							
1	Flour, plain, white	0	14.0	1450	341	9.4	1.3	0.2
2	Flour, wholemeal	0	14.0	1318	310	12.7	2.2	0.3
3	Oats, porridge, raw	0	8.2	1587	375	11.2	9.2	1.6
4	Rice, brown, boiled	0	66.0	597	141	2.6	1.1	0.3
5	Rice, white, boiled	0	68.0	587	138	2.6	1.3	0.3
6	Spaghetti, white, boiled	0	73.8	442	104	3.6	0.7	0.1
	Breads							
7	Brown bread, average	0	39.5	927	218	8.5	2.0	0.4
8	White bread, average	0	37.3	1002	235	8.4	1.9	0.4
9	White bread 'with added fibre' (soft grain)	0	40.0	978	230	7.6	1.5	0.4
10	Wholemeal bread, average	0	38.3	914	215	9.2	2.5	0.5
	Breakfast cereals							
11	Bran flakes	0	3.0	1353	318	10.2	1.9	0.4
12	Corn flakes	0	3.0	1535	360	7.9	0.7	0.1
13	Muesli, Swiss style	0	7.2	1540	363	9.8	5.9	0.8
14	Weetabix	0	5.6	1498	352	11.0	2.7	0.4
	Biscuits							
15	Chocolate biscuits, full coated	0	2.2	2197	524	5.7	27.6	16.7
16	Cream crackers	0	4.3	1857	440	9.5	16.3	N
17	Crispbread, rye	0	6.4	1367	321	9.4	2.1	0.3
18	Digestive biscuits, plain	0	2.5	1978	471	6.3	20.9	8.6
19	Semi-sweet biscuits	0	2.5	1925	457	6.7	16.6	8.0
	Buns and cakes							
20	Currant buns	0	27.7	1250	296	7.6	7.5	N
21	Fruit cake, rich	0	17.6	1438	341	3.8	11.0	3.4
22	Jam tarts, retail	0	14.4	1551	368	3.3	13.0	4.8
23	Madeira cake	0	20.2	1652	393	5.4	16.9	8.8
24	Swiss rolls, chocolate, individual	0	17.5	1421	337	4.3	11.3	N
	Puddings							
25	Bread pudding	0	29.3	1252	297	5.9	9.6	5.9
26	Cheesecake, frozen	0	44.0	1017	242	5.7	10.6	5.6
27	Custard made up with whole milk	0	75.5	495	117	3.7	4.5	2.8
28	Fruit crumble	0	54.8	835	198	2.0	6.9	2.1
29	Fruit pie, pastry top and bottom	0	47.9	1089	260	3.0	13.3	4.8
30	Rice pudding, canned	0	77.6	374	89	3.4	2.5	1.6
31	Trifle	0	67.2	674	160	3.6	6.3	3.1

Carbo-hydrate (g)	Total sugars (g)	Fibre NSP (g)	Calcium (mg)	Iron (mg)	Sodium (mg)	Vitamin A (µg)	Thiamin (mg)	Vitamin C (mg)	No.
77.7	1.5	3.1	140	2.0	3	0	0.31	0	1
63.9	2.1	9.0	38	3.9	3	0	0.47	0	2
66.0	1.1	7.1	52	3.8	9	0	0.90	0	3
32.1	0.5	0.8	4	0.5	1	0	0.14	0	4
30.9	0.0	0.1	18	0.2	1	0	0.01	0	5
22.2	0.5	1.2	7	0.5	0	0	0.01	0	6
44.3	3.0	3.5	100	2.2	540	0	0.27	0	7
49.3	2.6	1.5	110	1.6	520	0	0.21	0	8
49.6	3.3	3.1	150	2.3	450	0	0.20	0	9
41.6	1.8	5.8	54	2.7	550	0	0.34	0	10
69.3	18.7	13.0	50	20.0	1000	0	1.0	25	11
85.9	8.2	0.9	15	6.7	1110	0	1.0	0	12
72.2	26.2	6.4	110	5.8	380	0	0.5	0	13
75.7	5.2	9.7	35	7.4	270	0	0.9	0	14
67.4	43.4	2.1	110	1.7	160	0	0.03	0	15
68.3	0.0	2.2	110	1.7	610	0	0.23	0	16
70.6	3.2	11.7	45	3.5	220	0	0.28	0	17
68.6	13.6	2.2	92	3.2	600	0	0.14	0	18
74.8	22.3	1.7	120	2.1	410	0	0.13	0	19
52.7	15.1	N	110	1.9	230	N	0.37	0	20
59.6	48.4	1.7	82	1.9	200	125	0.08	0	21
63.4	36.0	N	72	1.7	130	N	0.06	0	22
58.4	36.5	0.9	42	1.1	380	N	0.06	0	23
58.1	41.8	N	77	1.1	350	N	0.12	0	24
49.7	33.1	1.2	120	1.6	310	107	0.10	0	25
33.0	22.2	0.9	68	0.5	160	N	0.04	0	26
16.6	11.4	0.0	130	0.1	81	63	0.04	1	27
34.0	21.3	1.7	49	0.6	68	88	0.05	3	28
34.0	12.0	1.8	59	0.8	200	74	0.08	3	29
14.0	8.2	0.2	93	0.2	50	N	0.03	0	30
22.3	16.8	0.5	79	0.5	53	75	0.06	4	31

Table 3.1. Composition per 100 g of edible portion (continued).

No.	Food	Inedible waste (%)	Water (g)	Energy (kJ)	Energy (kcal)	Protein (g)	Fat (g)	Saturated fatty acids (g)
	Milk and milk products							
32	Cream, fresh, single	0	73.7	817	198	2.6	19.1	11.9
33	Cream, fresh, double	0	47.5	1849	449	1.7	48.0	30.0
34	Dried skimmed milk	0	3.0	1482	348	36.1	0.6	0.4
35	Evaporated milk, whole	0	69.1	629	151	8.4	9.4	5.9
36	Ice cream, non-dairy, vanilla	0	65.3	746	178	3.2	8.7	4.4
37	Semi-skimmed milk, average	0	89.8	195	46	3.3	1.6	1.0
38	Skimmed milk, average	0	91.1	140	33	3.3	0.1	0.1
39	Whole milk, average	0	87.8	275	66	3.2	3.9	2.4
40	Yogurt, whole milk, plain	0	81.9	333	79	5.7	3.0	1.7
41	Yogurt, whole milk, fruit ('thick and creamy')	0	73.1	441	105	5.1	2.8	1.5
42	Yogurt, low fat, fruit	0	77.0	382	90	4.1	0.7	0.4
	Cheese							
43	Brie	0	48.6	1323	319	19.3	26.9	16.8
44	Cheddar, average	0	36.0	1708	412	25.5	34.4	21.7
45	Cheese spread, plain	0	53.3	1143	276	13.5	22.8	14.3
46	Cottage cheese, plain	0	79.1	413	98	13.8	3.9	2.4
47	Feta	0	56.5	1037	250	15.6	20.2	13.7
48	Fromage frais, fruit	0	71.9	551	131	6.8	5.8	3.6
	Eggs							
49	Eggs, chicken, boiled	0	75.1	612	147	12.5	10.8	3.1
50	Eggs, chicken, fried in vegetable oil	0	70.1	745	179	13.6	13.9	4.0
	Fats and oils							
51	Butter	0	15.6	3031	737	0.5	81.7	54.0
52	Low-fat spread	0	49.9	1605	390	5.8	40.5	11.2
53	Margarine, polyunsaturated	0	16.0	3039	739	0.2	81.6	16.2
54	Sunflower seed oil	0	0.0	3696	899	0.0	99.9	11.9
	Meat and meat products							
55	Bacon, rasher, lean and fat, raw back	6	40.5	1766	428	14.2	41.2	16.2
56	Bacon, rasher, lean and fat, grilled, back	0	36.0	1681	405	25.3	33.8	13.2
57	Beef, lean only, raw, average	0	74.0	517	123	20.3	4.6	1.9
58	Beef, mince, stewed	0	59.1	955	229	23.1	15.2	6.5
59	Beef, stewing steak, lean and fat, raw	4	68.7	736	176	20.2	10.6	4.5
60	Beef, stewing steak, lean and fat, stewed	0	57.1	932	223	30.9	11.0	4.7
61	Beefburgers, frozen, fried	0	53.0	1099	264	20.4	17.3	8.0
62	Black pudding, fried	0	44.0	1270	305	12.9	21.9	8.5

Carbo-hydrate (g)	Total sugars (g)	Fibre NSP (g)	Calcium (mg)	Iron (mg)	Sodium (mg)	Vitamin A (µg)	Thiamin (mg)	Vitamin C (mg)	No.
4.1	4.1	0.0	91	0.1	49	336	0.04	1	32
2.7	2.7	0.0	50	0.2	37	654	0.02	1	33
52.9	52.9	0.0	1280	0.27	550	351	0.38	13	34
8.5	8.5	0.0	290	0.26	180	122	0.07	1	35
23.1	19.2	0.0	120	0.1	76	2	0.04	1	36
5.0	5.0	0.0	120	0.05	55	23	0.04	1	37
5.0	5.0	0.0	120	0.06	54	1	0.04	1	38
4.8	4.8	0.0	115	0.06	55	55	0.03	1	39
7.8	7.8	N	200	0.01	80	31	0.06	1	40
15.7	15.7	N	160	0	82	42	0.06	1	41
17.9	17.9	N	150	0.1	64	11	0.05	1	42
0.0	0.0	0.0	540	0.8	700	320	0.04	0	43
0.1	0.1	0.0	720	0.3	670	363	0.03	0	44
4.4	4.4	0.0	420	0.2	1060	293	0.05	0	45
2.1	2.1	0.0	73	0.1	380	46	0.03	0	46
1.5	1.5	0.0	360	0.2	1440	225	0.04	0	47
13.8	13.8	0.0	86	0.1	35	N	0.02	0	48
0.0	0.0	0.0	57	1.9	140	190	0.07	0	49
0.0	0.0	0.0	65	2.2	160	215	0.07	0	50
0.0	0.0	0.0	15	0.2	750	887	0.00	0	51
0.5	0.5	0.0	39	0.0	650	501	0.00	0	52
1.0	1.0	0.0	4	0.3	800	946	0.00	0	53
0.0	0.0	0.0	0	0.0	0	0	0.00	0	54
0.0	0.0	0.0	7	1.0	1470	0	0.35	0	55
0.0	0.0	0.0	12	1.5	2020	0	0.43	0	56
0.0	0.0	0.0	7	2.1	61	0	0.07	0	57
0.0	0.0	0.0	18	3.1	320	0	0.05	0	58
0.0	0.0	0.0	8	2.1	72	0	0.06	0	59
0.0	0.0	0.0	15	3.0	360	0	0.03	0	60
7.0	1.4	N	33	3.1	880	0	0.02	0	61
15.0	0.0	N	35	20.0	1210	41	0.09	0	62

Table 3.1. Composition per 100 g of edible portion (continued).

No.	Food	Inedible waste (%)	Water (g)	Energy (kJ)	Energy (kcal)	Protein (g)	Fat (g)	Saturated fatty acids (g)
63	Bolognese sauce	0	74.7	602	145	8.0	11.1	3.1
64	Chicken, raw, meat and skin	36	64.4	954	230	17.6	17.7	5.9
65	Chicken, roast, meat only	0	68.4	621	148	24.8	5.4	1.6
66	Chicken, roast, meat and skin	0	61.9	902	216	22.6	14.0	4.2
67	Corned beef, canned	0	58.5	905	217	26.9	12.1	6.3
68	Ham, canned	0	72.5	502	120	18.4	5.1	1.9
69	Kidney, pig, raw	10	78.8	377	90	16.3	2.7	0.9
70	Kidney, pig, stewed	0	66.3	641	153	24.4	6.1	2.0
71	Lamb, lean only, raw, average	0	70.1	679	162	20.8	8.8	4.2
72	Lamb, roast, meat only	0	55.3	1106	266	26.1	17.9	8.9
73	Liver, lamb, raw	0	67.3	748	179	20.1	10.3	2.9
74	Liver, lamb, fried	0	58.4	970	232	22.9	14.0	4.0
75	Paté, liver	0	50.6	1308	316	13.1	28.9	8.4
76	Pork, lean only, raw, average	0	71.5	615	147	20.7	7.1	2.5
77	Pork chops, loin, lean only, grilled	0	56.1	945	226	32.3	10.7	3.8
78	Salami	0	28.0	2031	491	19.3	45.2	N
79	Sausages, beef, grilled	0	47.9	1104	265	13.0	17.3	6.7
80	Sausages, pork, grilled	0	45.1	1320	318	13.3	24.6	9.5
81	Sausages, low fat, grilled	0	50.1	959	229	16.2	13.8	5.0
82	Steak and kidney pie, individual	0	42.6	1349	323	9.1	21.2	8.4
83	Turkey, roast, meat and skin	0	65.0	717	171	28.0	6.5	2.1
	Fish and fish products							
84	Cod in batter, fried in blended oil	0	60.9	834	199	19.6	10.3	0.9
85	Fish fingers, grilled	0	56.2	899	214	15.1	9.0	2.8
86	Haddock, steamed, flesh only	24	75.1	417	98	22.8	0.8	0.2
87	Herring, grilled	0	65.5	828	199	20.4	13.0	3.7
88	Mackerel, fried	0	65.6	784	188	21.5	11.3	2.3
89	Pilchards, canned in tomato sauce	0	70.0	531	126	18.8	5.4	1.1
90	Prawns, boiled	0	70.0	451	107	22.6	1.8	0.4
91	Sardines, canned in oil, drained	17	58.4	906	217	23.7	13.6	2.8
92	Tuna, canned in brine, drained	19	74.6	422	99	23.5	0.6	0.2
	Potatoes and potato products							
93	Chips, homemade, fried in blended oil	0	56.5	796	189	3.9	6.7	0.6
94	Oven chips, frozen, baked	0	58.5	687	162	3.2	4.2	1.8
95	Potato crisps	0	1.9	2275	546	5.6	37.6	9.2
96	Potatoes, new, average, raw, flesh only	11	81.7	298	70	1.7	0.3	0.1
97	Potatoes, old, average, raw, flesh only	20	79.0	318	75	2.1	0.2	0.0
98	Potatoes, old, baked, flesh and skin	0	62.6	581	136	3.9	0.2	0.0

Carbo-hydrate (g)	Total sugars (g)	Fibre NSP (g)	Calcium (mg)	Iron (mg)	Sodium (mg)	Vitamin A (µg)	Thiamin (mg)	Vitamin C (mg)	No.
3.7	3.3	1.0	23	1.4	430	213	0.07	4	63
0	0.0	0.0	10	0.7	70	0	0.08	0	64
0.0	0.0	0.0	9	0.8	81	0	0.08	0	65
0.0	0.0	0.0	9	0.8	72	0	N	0	66
0.0	0.0	0.0	14	2.9	950	0	0.00	0	67
0.0	0.0	0.0	9	1.2	1250	0	0.52	0	68
0.0	0.0	0.0	8	5.0	190	160	0.32	14	69
0.0	0.0	0.0	13	6.4	370	46	0.19	11	70
0.0	0.0	0.0	7	1.6	88	0	0.14	0	71
0.0	0.0	0.0	8	2.5	65	0	0.12	0	72
1.6	0.0	0.0	7	9.4	76	38644	0.27	10	73
3.9	0.0	0.1	12	10.0	190	57300	0.26	12	74
1.0	0.3	0.0	15	7.1	790	7352	0.13	N	75
0.0	0.0	0.0	8	0.9	76	0	0.89	0	76
0.0	0.0	0.0	9	1.2	84	0	0.88	0	77
1.9	0.0	0.1	10	1.0	1850	0	0.21	N	78
15.2	2.4	0.7	73	1.7	1100	0	0.00	N	79
11.5	1.8	0.7	53	1.5	1000	0	0.02	N	80
10.8	0.9	1.5	130	1.3	1190	0	0.00	N	81
25.6	2.3	0.9	53	2.5	510	N	0.12	0	82
0.0	0.0	0.0	9	0.9	52	N	N	0	83
7.5	0.1	0.3	80	0.5	100	N	0.20	0	84
19.3	0.0	0.7	52	0.8	380	0	0.10	0	85
0.0	0.0	0.0	55	0.7	120	0	0.08	0	86
0.0	0.0	0.0	33	1.0	170	34	0.00	0	87
0.0	0.0	0.0	28	1.2	150	43	0.09	0	88
0.7	0.6	0.0	300	2.7	370	32	0.02	0	89
0.0	0.0	0.0	150	1.1	1590	0	0.02	0	90
0.0	0.0	0.0	550	2.9	650	11	0.04	0	91
0.0	0.0	0.0	8	1.0	320	N	0.02	0	92
30.1	0.6	2.2	11	0.8	12	0	0.24	9	93
29.8	0.7	2.0	12	0.8	53	0	0.11	12	94
49.3	0.7	4.9	37	1.8	1070	0	0.11	27	95
16.1	1.3	1.0	6	0.3	11	0	0.15	16	96
17.2	0.6	1.3	5	0.4	7	0	0.21	11	97
31.7	1.2	2.7	11	0.7	12	0	0.37	14	98

Table 3.1. Composition per 100 g of edible portion (continued).

No.	Food	Inedible waste (%)	Water (g)	Energy (kJ)	Energy (kcal)	Protein (g)	Fat (g)	Saturated fatty acids (g)
99	Potatoes, old, boiled in unsalted water	0	80.3	306	72	1.8	0.1	0.0
100	Potatoes, old, roast in blended oil	0	64.7	630	149	2.9	4.5	0.4
	Vegetables							
101	Aubergine, raw	4	92.9	64	15	0.9	0.4	0.1
102	Beans, baked, canned in tomato sauce	0	71.5	355	84	5.2	0.6	0.1
103	Beans, red kidney, canned, drained	36	67.5	424	100	6.9	0.6	0.1
104	Beans, runner, boiled in unsalted water	0	92.8	76	18	1.2	0.5	0.1
105	Beetroot, boiled in salted water	20	82.4	195	46	2.3	0.1	0.0
106	Brussels sprouts, boiled in unsalted water	0	86.9	153	35	2.9	1.3	0.3
107	Cabbage, raw, average	23	90.1	109	26	1.7	0.4	0.1
108	Cabbage, boiled in unsalted water, average	0	93.1	67	16	1.0	0.4	0.1
109	Carrots, old, boiled in unsalted water	0	90.5	100	24	0.6	0.4	0.1
110	Cauliflower, boiled in unsalted water	0	90.6	117	28	2.9	0.9	0.2
111	Celery, raw	9	95.1	32	7	0.5	0.2	0.0
112	Courgette, raw	12	93.7	74	18	1.8	0.4	0.1
113	Cucumber	3	96.4	40	10	0.7	0.1	0.0
114	Lentils, (red, dried) boiled in unsalted water	0	72.1	424	100	7.6	0.4	0.0
115	Lettuce, average	26	95.1	59	14	0.8	0.5	0.1
116	Mycoprotein, Quorn	0	75.0	360	86	11.8	3.5	0.6
117	Mushrooms, raw	3	92.6	55	13	1.8	0.5	0.1
118	Onions, raw	9	89.0	150	36	1.2	0.2	0.0
119	Parsnips, boiled in unsalted water	0	78.7	278	66	1.6	1.2	0.2
120	Peas, frozen, boiled in unsalted water	0	78.3	291	69	6.0	0.9	0.2
121	Peppers (green, raw)	16	93.3	65	15	0.8	0.3	0.1
122	Plantain, boiled in unsalted water	0	68.5	477	112	0.8	0.2	0.1
123	Processed peas, canned, re-heated, drained	35	69.6	423	99	6.9	0.7	0.1
124	Spinach, frozen, boiled in unsalted water	0	91.6	90	21	3.1	0.8	0.1
125	Sweetpotato, boiled in salted water	0	74.7	358	84	1.1	0.3	0.1
126	Sweetcorn kernels, canned, re-heated, drained	18	72.3	519	122	2.9	1.2	0.2
127	Tofu, soya bean, steamed	0	85.0	304	73	8.1	4.2	0.5
128	Tomatoes, raw	0	93.1	73	17	0.7	0.3	0.1
129	Turnip, boiled in unsalted water	0	93.1	51	12	0.6	0.2	0.0

Carbo-hydrate (g)	Total sugars (g)	Fibre NSP (g)	Calcium (mg)	Iron (mg)	Sodium (mg)	Vitamin A (µg)	Thiamin (mg)	Vitamin C (mg)	No.
17.0	0.7	1.2	5	0.4	7	0	0.18	6	99
25.9	0.6	1.8	8	0.7	9	0	0.23	8	100
2.2	2.0	2.0	10	0.3	2	12	0.02	4	101
15.3	5.9	3.7	53	1.4	530	12	0.09	0	102
17.8	3.6	6.2	71	2.0	390	1	0.21	0	103
2.3	2.0	1.9	22	1.0	1	20	0.05	10	104
9.5	8.8	1.9	29	0.8	110	5	0.01	5	105
3.5	3.0	3.1	20	0.5	2	53	0.07	60	106
4.1	4.0	2.4	52	0.7	5	64	0.15	49	107
2.2	2.0	1.8	33	0.3	8	35	0.08	20	108
4.9	4.6	2.5	24	0.4	50	1260	0.09	2	109
2.1	1.8	1.6	17	0.4	4	10	0.07	27	110
0.9	0.9	1.1	41	0.4	60	8	0.06	8	111
1.8	1.7	0.9	25	0.8	1	100	0.12	21	112
1.5	1.4	0.6	18	0.3	3	10	0.03	2	113
17.5	0.8	1.9	16	2.4	12	3	0.11	0	114
1.7	1.7	0.9	28	0.7	3	59	0.12	5	115
2.0	1.1	4.8	N	N	240	0	36.6	0	116
0.4	0.2	1.1	6	0.6	5	0	0.09	1	117
7.9	5.6	1.4	25	0.3	3	2	0.13	5	118
12.9	5.9	4.7	50	0.6	4	5	0.07	10	119
9.7	2.7	5.1	35	1.6	2	67	0.26	12	120
2.6	2.4	1.6	8	0.4	4	44	0.01	120	121
28.5	5.5	1.2	5	0.5	4	58	0.03	9	122
17.5	1.5	4.8	33	1.8	380	10	0.10	0	123
0.5	0.3	2.1	150	1.7	16	640	0.06	6	124
20.5	11.6	2.3	23	0.7	32	660	0.07	17	125
26.6	9.6	1.4	4	0.5	270	19	0.04	1	126
0.7	0.3	N	510	1.2	4	0	0.06	0	127
3.1	3.1	1.0	7	0.5	9	105	0.09	17	128
2.0	1.9	1.9	45	0.2	28	3	0.05	10	129

Table 3.1. Composition per 100 g of edible portion (continued).

No.	Food	Inedible waste (%)	Water (g)	Energy (kJ)	Energy (kcal)	Protein (g)	Fat (g)	Saturated fatty acids (g)
130	Watercress	38	92.5	94	22	3.0	1.0	0.3
131	Yam, boiled in unsalted water	0	64.4	568	133	1.7	0.3	0.1
	Fruit							
132	Apples, eating, average, raw, flesh and skin	11	84.5	199	47	0.4	0.1	0.0
133	Apricots, ready-to-eat	0	29.7	674	158	4.0	0.6	N
134	Apricots, canned in syrup	0	80.0	268	63	0.4	0.1	0.0
135	Avocado, average, flesh only	29	72.5	784	190	1.9	19.5	4.1
136	Bananas, flesh only	34	75.1	403	95	1.2	0.3	0.1
137	Blackcurrants, stewed, without sugar	0	80.7	103	24	0.8	0.0	0.0
138	Cherries, raw, weighed without stones	17	82.8	203	48	0.9	0.1	0.0
139	Dates, dried, weighed without stones	16	14.6	1151	270	3.3	0.2	0.1
140	Figs, dried, ready to eat	0	23.6	889	209	3.3	1.5	N
141	Gooseberries, cooking, stewed without sugar	0	78.9	310	73	0.4	0.2	N
142	Grapefruit, raw, flesh only	32	89.0	126	30	0.8	0.1	0.0
143	Grapes, seedless	5	81.8	257	60	0.4	0.1	0.0
144	Kiwi fruit, flesh and seeds	14	84.0	207	49	1.1	0.5	N
145	Mangoes, ripe, raw, flesh only	32	82.4	245	57	0.7	0.2	0.1
146	Melon, honeydew, flesh only	37	92.2	119	28	0.6	0.1	0.0
147	Oranges, flesh only	30	86.1	158	37	1.1	0.1	0.0
148	Peaches, raw, flesh and skin	10	88.9	142	33	1.0	0.1	
149	Peaches, canned in syrup	0	81.1	233	55	0.5	0.0	0.0
150	Pears, average, raw, flesh and skin	9	83.8	169	40	0.3	0.1	0.0
151	Pineapple, canned in juice	0	86.8	200	47	0.3	0.0	0.0
152	Plums, average, raw, flesh and skin	6	83.9	155	36	0.6	0.1	0.0
153	Prunes, ready-to-eat	0	31.1	601	141	2.5	0.4	N
154	Raspberries, raw	0	87.0	109	25	1.4	0.3	0.1
155	Rhubarb, stewed with sugar	0	84.6	203	48	0.9	0.1	0.0
156	Strawberries, raw	5	89.5	113	27	0.8	0.1	0.0
157	Sultanas	0	15.2	1171	275	2.7	0.4	N
	Nuts							
158	Almonds, flesh only	63	4.2	2534	612	21.1	55.8	4.7
159	Coconut, desiccated	0	2.3	2492	604	5.6	62.0	53.4
160	Peanut butter, smooth	0	1.1	2581	623	22.6	53.7	11.7
161	Peanuts, roasted and salted	0	1.9	2491	602	24.5	53.0	9.5
	Sugars and preserves							
162	Chocolate, milk	0	2.2	2214	529	8.4	30.3	17.8
163	Honey	0	23.0	1229	288	0.4	0.0	0.0

Carbo-hydrate (g)	Total sugars (g)	Fibre NSP (g)	Calcium (mg)	Iron (mg)	Sodium (mg)	Vitamin A (µg)	Thiamin (mg)	Vitamin C (mg)	No.
0.4	0.4	1.5	170	2.2	49	420	0.16	62	130
33.0	0.7	1.4	12	0.4	17	0	0.14	4	131
11.8	11.8	1.8	4	0.1	3	3	0.03	6	132
36.5	36.5	6.3	73	3.4	14	91	0.00	1	133
16.1	16.1	0.9	19	0.2	10	25	0.01	5	134
1.9	0.5	3.4	11	0.4	6	3	0.10	6	135
23.2	20.9	1.1	6	0.3	1	3	0.04	11	136
5.6	5.6	3.1	51	1.1	2	14	0.02	130	137
11.5	11.5	0.9	13	0.2	1	4	0.03	11	138
68.0	68.0	4.0	45	1.3	10	7	0.07	0	139
48.6	48.6	6.9	230	3.9	57	10	0.07	1	140
18.5	2.5	2.0	23	0.3	2	7	0.01	11	141
6.8	6.8	1.3	23	0.1	3	3	0.05	36	142
15.4	15.4	0.7	13	0.3	2	3	0.05	3	143
10.6	10.3	1.9	25	0.4	4	6	0.01	59	144
14.1	13.8	2.6	12	0.7	2	300	0.04	37	145
6.6	6.6	0.6	9	0.1	32	8	0.03	9	146
8.5	8.5	1.7	47	0.1	5	5	0.11	54	147
									148
14.0	14.0	0.9	3	0.2	4	13	0.01	5	149
10.0	10.0	2.2	11	0.2	3	3	0.02	6	150
12.2	12.2	0.5	8	0.5	1	2	0.09	11	151
8.8	8.8	1.6	13	0.4	2	49	0.05	4	152
34.0	34.0	5.7	34	2.6	11	23	0.09	0	153
4.6	4.6	2.5	25	0.7	3	1	0.03	32	154
11.5	11.5	1.2	33	0.1	1	5	0.03	5	155
6.0	6.0	1.1	16	0.4	6	1	0.03	77	156
69.4	69.4	2.0	64	2.2	19	2	0.09	0	157
6.9	4.2	7.4	240	3.0	14	0	0.21	0	158
6.4	6.4	13.7	23	3.6	28	0	0.03	0	159
13.1	6.7	5.4	37	2.1	350	0	0.17	0	160
7.1	3.8	6.0	37	1.3	400	0	0.18	0	161
59.4	56.5	0.0	220	1.6	120	7	0.1	0	162
76.4	76.4	0.0	5	0.4	11	0	0.0	0	163

Table 3.1. Composition per 100 g of edible portion (continued).

No.	Food	Inedible waste (%)	Water (g)	Energy (kJ)	Energy (kcal)	Protein (g)	Fat (g)	Saturated fatty acids (g)
164	Jam, fruit with edible seeds	0	29.8	1114	261	0.6	0.0	0.0
165	Marmalade	0	28.0	1114	261	0.1	0.0	0.0
166	Peppermints	0	0.2	1670	392	0.5	0.7	N
167	Sugar, white	0	0.0	1680	394	0.0	0.0	0.0
168	Syrup, golden	0	20.0	1269	298	0.3	0.0	0.0
	Beverages							
169	Cocoa powder	0	3.4	1301	312	18.5	21.7	12.8
170	Coffee, infusion, 5 minutes	0	N	8	2	0.2	0.0	0.0
171	Coffee, instant powder	0	3.4	424	100	14.6	0.0	0.0
172	Drinking chocolate powder	0	2.1	1554	366	5.5	6.0	3.5
173	Tea, Indian, infusion	0	N	2	0	0.1	0.0	0.0
	Soft drinks and juices							
174	Coca-cola	0	89.8	168	39	0.0	0.0	0.0
175	Lemonade, bottled	0	94.6	90	21	0.0	0.0	0.0
176	Orange drink, undiluted	0	71.2	456	107	0.0	0.0	0.0
177	Orange juice, unsweetened	0	89.2	153	36	0.5	0.1	0.0
178	Pineapple juice, unsweetened	0	87.8	177	41	0.3	0.1	0
	Miscellaneous							
179	Baking powder	0	6.3	693	163	5.2	0.0	0.0
180	Curry powder	0	8.5	979	233	9.5	10.8	N
181	Marmite	0	25.4	730	172	39.7	0.7	N
182	Mayonnaise, retail	0	18.8	2843	691	1.1	75.6	11.1
183	Mustard, smooth	0	63.7	579	139	7.1	8.2	0.5
184	Pickle, sweet	0	58.9	572	134	0.6	0.3	0.0
185	Salad cream	0	47.2	1440	348	1.5	31.0	3.9
186	Soup, cream of tomato, canned, ready to serve	0	84.2	230	55	0.8	3.3	N
187	Soy sauce	0	67.6	266	64	8.7	0.0	0.0
188	Tomato ketchup	0	64.8	420	98	2.1	0.0	0.0
	Composition per 100 ml							
	Alcoholic drinks							
189	Beer, bitter, keg	0	93.5	129	31	0.3	0.0	0.0
190	Cider, dry	0	93.2	152	36	0.0	0.0	0.0
191	Lager, bottled	0	94.9	120	29	0.2	0.0	0.0
192	Spirits, 40% volume	0	63.3	919	222	0.0	0.0	0.0
193	Wine, white, medium	0	86.3	311	75	0.1	0.0	0.0
194	Wine, red	0	88.0	284	68	0.2	0.0	0.0

N = not determined.

Carbo-hydrate (g)	Total sugars (g)	Fibre NSP (g)	Calcium (mg)	Iron (mg)	Sodium (mg)	Vitamin A (μg)	Thiamin (mg)	Vitamin C (mg)	No.
69.0	69.0	N	24	1.5	16	0	0.0	10	164
69.5	69.5	0.6	35	0.6	18	8	0.0	10	165
102.2	102.2	0.0	7	0.2	9	0	0.0	0	166
105.0	105.0	0.0	2	0.0	0	0	0.0	0	167
79.0	79.0	0.0	26	1.5	270	0	0.0	0	168
11.5	0.0	12.1	130	10.5	950	7	0.16	0	169
0.3	0.3	0.0	2	0.0	0	N	0.00	0	170
11.0	6.5	0.0	160	4.4	41	N	0.00	0	171
77.4	73.8	N	33	2.4	250	N	0.06	0	172
0.0	0.0	0.0	0	0.0	0	0	0.00	0	173
10.5	10.5	0.0	4	0.0	8	0	0.00	0	174
5.6	5.6	0.0	5	0.0	7	0	0.00	0	175
28.5	28.5	0.0	8	0.1	21	N	0.00	0	176
8.8	8.8	0.1	10	0.2	10	3	0.08	39	177
10.5	10.5	0.0	8	0.2	8	1	0.06	11	178
37.8	0.0	0.0	1130	0.0	11800	0	0.00	0	179
26.1	N	23.0	640	58.3	450	17	0.25	0	180
1.8	0.0	0.0	95	3.7	4500	0	3.10	0	181
1.7	1.3	0.0	8	0.3	450	103	0.02	N	182
9.7	7.8	N	70	2.9	2950	N	N	0	183
34.4	32.6	1.2	19	2.0	1700	42	0.03	0	184
16.7	16.7	N	18	0.5	1040	12	N	0	185
5.9	2.6	N	17	0.4	460	35	0.03	0	186
8.3	N	0.0	19	2.7	5720	0	0.05	0	187
24.0	22.9	0.9	25	1.2	1120	38	1.00	2	188
2.3	2.3	0.0	8	0.01	8	0	0	0	189
2.6	2.6	0.0	8	0.5	7	0	0	0	190
1.5	1.5	0.0	4	0.0	4	0	0	0	191
0.0	0.0	0.0	0	0.0	0	0	0	0	192
3.4	3.4	0.0	14	1.2	21	0	0	0	193
0.3	0.3	0.0	7	0.9	10	0	0	0	194

Appendix 4 The use of food tables for calculations of the nutritional value of foods

A great deal of useful information can be worked out from the food composition tables in Appendix 3. Examples of various types of calculations are given below:

1. NUTRIENT CONTENT

(a) *Simple nutrient content*

To calculate the protein content of 2 grilled fish fingers
Fish fingers (food no. 85) contain 15.1g protein per 100 g
2 fish fingers weigh 56 g (Appendix 5)

$$56 \text{ g grilled fish fingers contain } 15.1 \times \frac{56}{100}$$

$$= 8.5 \text{ g protein}$$

(b) *Nutrient content allowing for wastage (inedible matter)*

To calculate the carbohydrate content of one apple weighing 120 g:
Eating apples (food no. 132) contain 10.5 g carbohydrate per 100 g edible portion, and 11 per cent waste

$$\text{A 120-g apple contains } \frac{100 - 11}{100} \times 120 \text{ g edible matter}$$

$$= 106.8 \text{ g edible matter}$$

$$\text{Therefore 106.8 g (120-g whole apple) contains } 10.5 \times \frac{106.8}{100} \text{ g}$$

$$= 11.2 \text{ g carbohydrate}$$

2. PORTION SIZES

(a) *400 kJ portions*

Cheddar cheese, for example:
Cheddar cheese (food no. 44) has an energy value of 1708 kJ per 100 g

$$400 \text{ kJ are contained in } \frac{100}{1708} \times 400 = 23 \text{ g (a little less than 1 oz Cheddar cheese)}$$

or cottage cheese:

Cottage cheese (food no.46) has an energy value of 413 kJ per 100 g

400 kJ are contained in $\dfrac{100}{413} \times 400 = 97$ g (or 3½ oz) of cottage cheese

(b) *100-kcal portions* (the size of a 100-kcal portion will be slightly greater than a 400-kJ portion and slightly smaller than a 500-kJ portion)

Old potatoes, uncooked, for example:

Old potatoes (food no. 97) have an energy value of 75 kcal per 100 g edible portion

100 kcal are contained in $\dfrac{100}{75} \times 100 = 133$ g potato

Since the potatoes contain 20 per cent inedible material (peelings) this is equivalent to

$133 \times \dfrac{100}{100 - 20}$ g $= 166$ g whole potato

3. COST OF NUTRIENTS

(a) *Nutrients per penny*

To calculate the nutrients obtained per penny from a large (800 g) loaf of sliced wholemeal bread costing 65p:

1p buys $\dfrac{1}{65} \times 800 = 12.3$ g

Food no. 10 shows the nutrients in 100 g wholemeal bread. Therefore multiply the values for each nutrient by $\dfrac{12.3}{100}$ = 1.1 g protein

0.3 g fat

5.1 g carbohydrate

6.6 mg calcium

0.3 mg iron, etc.

(b) To calculate the cost of 10 g protein from *baked beans*

Baked beans (food no. 102) contain 5.2 g protein per 100 g

10 g protein are contained in $\dfrac{10}{5.2} \times 100 = 192.3$ g baked beans

At a cost of 28p per 450-g can

192.3 g of baked beans cost $\dfrac{192.3}{450} \times 28 = 12.0$ pence

4. PERCENTAGE OF ENERGY FROM FAT

(a) In a food such as brown bread:

Brown bread (food no. 7) contains 2.0 g fat and 927 kJ (218 kcal) per 100 g

Each gram of fat provides 37 kJ (9 kcal)

The percentage of energy from fat $= \dfrac{2.0 \times 37}{927} \times 100 = 8.0\%$

$$(\text{or } \dfrac{2.0 \times 9}{218} \times 100 = 8.3\%)$$

(b) Margarine:

Margarine (food no. 53) contains 81.6 g fat and 3039 kJ (739 kcal) per 100 g

Each gram of fat provides 37 kJ (9 kcal)

The percentage of energy from fat $= \dfrac{81.6 \times 37}{3039} \times 100 = 99.4\%$

$$(\text{or } \dfrac{81.6 \times 9}{739} \times 100 = 99.4\%)$$

(c) In a combination of foods:

One slice of brown bread weighs 30 g and 7 g of margarine is allowed for spreading on one slice.

One slice (30 g) brown bread contains

$(2.0 \times \dfrac{30}{100})$ g fat and $(927 \times \dfrac{30}{100})$kJ

$= 0.6$ g fat and 278.1 kJ (65.4 kcal)

7 g margarine contains $(81.6 \times \dfrac{7}{100})$ g fat and $(3039 \times \dfrac{7}{100})$ kJ

$= 5.7$ g fat and 212.7 kJ (51.7 kcal)

The combination slice of bread with margarine contains 0.6 + 5.7 g fat = 6.3 g fat and 278.1 + 212.7 kJ = 490.8 kJ (117.1 kcal)

Since each gram of fat provides 37 kJ or 9 kcal, the percentage of energy from fat in a slice of bread and butter is

$$\frac{6.3 \times 37 \times 100}{490.8} = 47.5\%$$

$$(\text{or } \frac{6.3 \times 9 \times 100}{117.1} = 48.4\%)$$

Adding baked beans, a banana, jam or a drink such as fruit juice would further reduce the proportion of energy derived from fat.

N.B. The values derived from kilojoules and kilocalories differ slightly since the conversion factors given on p. 128 are not exactly equivalent.

Appendix 5 Approximate servings of commonly used foods

Milk, whole	for 1 cup of tea/coffee	25 g
Milk, semi-skimmed }	for 1 cup of tea/coffee	30 g
	for 1 glass	200 g
Cheese, Cheddar type	'matchbox-sized' piece	30 g
Chicken, roast	medium average portion	100 g
Pork chop	medium size, with bone, grilled	150 g
Minced beef	medium average portion, cooked	140 g
Bacon	rasher, average, fried/grilled	40 g
Sausage	large sausage, cooked	40 g
Meat pie	individual pie	150 g
Beefburger, 100% beef	1 burger, fried/grilled	34 g
Fish finger	1 fish finger, grilled	28 g
Tuna	1 portion for sandwich	45 g
Egg	size 3, no shell	57 g
Butter, margarine or low-fat spread	for 1 slice bread	7–10 g
Peanut butter	thickly spread on 1 slice	20 g
Jam or marmalade	average spreading on 1 slice	15 g
Lettuce	average serving in salad	30 g
Tomato	1 slice	17 g
Potatoes, boiled	1 average portion, medium	175 g
mashed	1 scoop	60 g
Chips	medium portion	165 g
Peas	medium portion	70 g
Orange	medium-sized (without peel)	160 g
Apple	medium-sized, eating	112 g
Banana	1 medium without skin	100 g
Fruit juice	average glass	160 g
Bread white, small loaf	slice	25 g
Bread white, large loaf	medium slice	36 g
Bread wholemeal, small loaf	slice	25 g

Bread wholemeal, large loaf	medium slice	36 g
Flour	1 tablespoon, rounded	30 g
Porridge	medium portion	160 g
Breakfast cereal	cornflakes type, medium helping	30 g
Crispbread	1 crispbread, wholemeal	15 g
Biscuits, digestive	1 biscuit	13 g
Rice	medium portion, boiled	180 g
Pasta	average medium portion, cooked	230 g
Coffee, instant	1 heaped teaspoon	2 g
Drinking chocolate	per mug	18 g
Sugar	1 level teaspoon	4 g
Beer	half pint	287 g (284 ml)
Wine	1 average wineglass	125 g (125 ml)

Appendix 6　The Balance of Good Health

The Balance of Good Health previously developed by the Health Education Authority, the Department of Health and the Ministry of Agriculture, Fisheries and Food and is based on the Government's Eight Guidelines for a Healthy Diet. It now forms the basis of the Food Standards Agency Nutrition Strategy.

- Enjoy your food
- Eat a variety of different foods
- Eat the right amount to be a healthy weight
- Eat plenty of foods rich in starch and fibre
- Eat plenty of fruit and vegetables
- Don't eat too many foods that contain a lot of fat
- Don't have sugary foods and drinks too often
- If you drink alcohol, drink sensibly

The Balance of Good Health illustrates these messages in graphic form (see illustration) by showing the types and proportions of foods needed to make up a well-balanced and healthy diet. The balance of foods to be achieved is shown by the different areas occupied by each of five food groups: *bread, other cereals and potatoes; fruit and vegetables; meat, fish and alternatives; milk and dairy foods;* and *fatty and sugary foods.* Choosing food groups in the approximate proportions shown and choosing different foods from within each group helps to ensure that all essential nutrients are consumed in adequate amounts. People differ in the amount of energy they need and hence in the amount of food they should eat, but whatever that may be the proportions of foods from the different groups should remain the same. It is not particularly important to achieve the balance shown at every meal, or even every day, although this is one approach. The balance can be achieved over the course of a week or two. The Guide applies to most people including people whose weight is in the desired range for their height, those who are overweight, vegetarians and people of all ethnic origins. It does not apply to children under two years of age who need full fat milk and dairy products. People under medical supervision or with special dietary requirements should check with their doctor to be clear whether the Guide applies to them.

A copy of *The Balance of Good Health* can be obtained from The Food Standards Agency Publication line on 0845 6060667. Further information is available from the FSA, 808c Aviation House, 125 Kingsway, London WC2B 6NH.

The Balance of Good Health

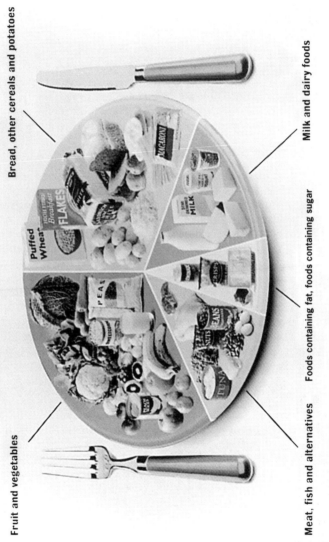
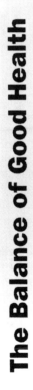

Fruit and vegetables

Bread, other cereals and potatoes

Milk and dairy foods

Foods containing fat, foods containing sugar

Meat, fish and alternatives

Appendix 7   Food additives

In addition to the expected ingredients of made-up foods there are other substances which may be added in small amounts to perform a special function in the food. These are called food additives. They fall into two broad categories: those which are added to prevent food spoilage and those which are added to enhance the texture, flavour or appearance of food.

Preservatives and antioxidants

It is very important that every effort is made to prevent sound food being wasted. Some forms of food spoilage, such as attacks on stored food by vermin, are easily recognised. Other forms of spoilage develop within the food itself and give rise to off-flavours long before the visual appearance of the food itself is noticeably affected; these may arise either by the action of micro-organisms (i.e. moulds and bacteria) or by chemical action. While some microorganisms merely make the food unpalatable, others such as *Clostridium botulinum* produce highly poisonous toxins and present a considerable hazard to health. Preservatives such as sulphur dioxide and sodium nitrite are added to some foods to inhibit the growth of microorganisms. The most common form of chemical spoilage is rancidity. Rancidity resulting from the oxidation of fat can be retarded by the addition of antioxidants. Some antioxidants are natural compounds but in order to protect fat in foods which are baked (e.g. biscuits), heat-stable synthetic antioxidants are required.

Other additives

The texture of food often depends on the ability of added emulsifiers to form a uniform dispersion of fat and water (as in margarine and salad cream). Similarly, stabilisers are added to prevent uniform dispersions separating out (for example, the setting of instant desserts).

The colour and flavour of foods are closely linked: consumers expect a food to have a colour which matches the flavour. Therefore, if the natural colour is lost or changed during processing, colouring matter may be added to restore the food to the expected colour.

The law strictly controls the types and quantities of additives which may be used in food (see also Appendix 8), and the list of ingredients must show the additive category name (e.g. colour), and the serial number of the additive or its name (e.g. E300 ascorbic acid, or E500 sodium bicarbonate) or both.

Appendix 8   Legislation governing the composition and labelling of food

The primary legislation in this field is the Food Safety Act 1990. This extends throughout Great Britain and similar legislation applies in Northern Ireland, the Channel Islands and Isle of Man.

The Act sets out a framework to protect consumers from food being sold which:

(a) is unsafe because it has been rendered injurious to health or is unfit or too contaminated for human consumption;

(b) is not of the nature, substance or quality demanded;

(c) is labelled, advertised or displayed in a manner which falsely describes or misleads.

These general provisions are backed up by many regulations which lay down detailed requirements as to the labelling of all foods, the composition of certain foods, and the type and level of additives and contaminants permitted in food (see below).

Food and Health Ministers are jointly responsible for making legislation. Ministers are advised on the need for and type of regulations by the Food Advisory Committee which may choose to consult all interested parties, including consumers, enforcement officers and the food industry before making any recommendations. However, the Ministers are required to consult organisations that are representative of interests likely to be affected by such legislative proposals.

The Food Labelling Regulations 1996 require most pre-packed foods to bear, amongst other things, its name, a list of ingredients (in descending order by ingoing weight), the name and address of the manufacturer or packer or seller established within the EU and the appropriate indication of durability (a 'sell by' or 'best before' date mark) and they include rules on nutrition labelling. These regulations also set conditions for claiming that a food has certain properties (for example, that it is a source of specified vitamins and minerals). Nurtrition labelling is compulsory when a nutrition claim (e.g. 'low fat', 'high fibre') is made, otherwise it can be given voluntarily. When nutrition labelling is given, labels must at the minimum show the amount of energy, protein, carbohydrate and fat provided by 100 g or 100 ml of the food. Per serving or per portion information may be given as well. Some labels show a second group of nutrients which include sugars (as part of carbohydrates), saturates (as part of fat), fibre and sodium. All of the second group have to be added to the basic list if a manufacturer lists or makes a claim about any of them. Labels can also show the amount of polyols (as parts of carbohydrate), starches, monounsaturates, polyunsaturates and cholesterol (as parts of fat) and the amount and percentage of the labellling RDA (a single value is set for food labelling purposes which is sufficient for the needs of the population as a whole) of certain vitamins and minerals provided the food contains a significant amount. Nutrition information must include the amount of any nutrient if a claim is made about it, including any not already mentioned.

Compositional regulations lay down standards for certain foods. For example minimum meat contents are linked to certain permitted names in the Meat Products Regulations. A pork sausage, for instance, under the Meat Products and Spreadable Fish Products Regulations 1984 must contain 65 per cent meat but a beef sausage only 50 per cent.

Certain requirements for the composition of bread are laid down by the Bread and Flour Regulations 1998. The Regulations restrict the use of specified ingredients which may be used in the preparation of flour and bread. The Regulations prescribe the levels of added calcium, iron, thiamin and nicotinic acid required in flour.

The Spreadable Fats (Marketing Standards) Regulations 1995 (as amended) lay down compositional, labelling and marketing standards for spreadable fats (butter, margarine, mixtures and reduced fat spreads) including fortification requirements for vitamins A and D in margarine.

These are also regulations which lay down lists of permitted additives and standards of purity. The safety of additives and the need for their use are given full and detailed consideration before they are permitted to be used in food. Existing regulations control, for example, preservatives, sweeteners, colourings, antioxidants, and emulsifiers and stabilisers. Food contaminants such as heavy metals are also controlled by legislation.

Appendix 9   Books for further reading

Department of Health. *Feeding today's infants.* London: HMSO, 1988 (ISBN 0 11 321181 3).

Department of Health. *The diets of British school children.* Report on health and social subjects No. 36. London: HMSO, 1989 (ISBN 0 11 321223 2).

Department of Health. *Dietary sugars and human disease.* Report on health and social subjects No. 37. London: HMSO, 1989 (0 11 321255 0).

Department of Health. *Dietary Reference Values for food energy and nutrients for the United Kingdom.* Report on health and social subjects No. 41. London: HMSO, 1991 (minor amendments, revised Chapter 36, 1994) (ISBN 0 11 321397 2).

Department of Health. *Dietary Reference Values: a guide.* London: HMSO, 1991 (ISBN 0 11 321396 4).

Department of Health. *The nutrition of elderly people.* Report on health and social subjects No. 43. London: HMSO, 1992 (ISBN 0 11 321550 9).

Department of Health. *The Health of the Nation. A summary of the strategy for health in England.* HMSO, 1992.

Department of Health. *Folic acid and the prevention of neural tube defects.* Heywood: Health Publications Unit, 1992.

Department of Health. *The nutritional assessment of novel foods and processes. Report of the Panel on Novel Foods of the Committee on Medical Aspects of Food Policy.* Report on health and social subjects No. 44. London: HMSO, 1993 (ISBN 0 11 321632 7).

Department of Health. *Weaning and the weaning diet.* Report on health and social subjects No. 45. London. HMSO, 1994 (ISBN 0 11 321838 9).

Department of Health. *Nutritional aspects of cardiovascular disease. Report of the Cardiovascular Review Group of the Committee on Medical Aspects of Food Policy.* Report on health and social subjects No. 46. London. HMSO, 1994 (ISBN 0 11 321875 3).

Department of Health. *Nutritional aspects of the development of cancer.* Report on health and social subjects No. 48. London, The Stationery Office, 1998 (ISBN 0 11 322089 8)

Department of Health. *Nutrition and bone health: with particular reference to calcium and vitamin D.* Report on health and social subjects No. 49. London, The Stationery Office, 1998 (ISBN 0 11 322262 9).

J C Drummond and A Wilbraham. *The Englishman's food*. London: Pimlico, 1991.

S Finch, W Doyle, C Lowe, C Bates, A Prentice, G Smithers, P Clarke. *National Diet and Nutrition Survey: people aged 65 years and over. Volume 1: Report of the diet and nutrition survey.* London: The Stationery Office, 1998 (ISBN 0 11 243019 8)

J S Garrow and W P T James (eds). *Human nutrition and dietetics*. 9th edition, Edinburgh: Churchill Livingstone, 1993 (ISBN 0 443 04121 0).

J Gregory, K Foster, H Tyler and M Wiseman. *The dietary and nutritional survey of British adults*. London: HMSO, 1990 (ISBN 0 11 691300 2).

J R Gregory, D L Collins, P S W Davies, J M Hughes and P C Clarke. *National Diet and Nutrition Survey: children aged 1½ to 4½ years. Volume 1: Report of the diet and nutrition survey.* London: HMSO, 1995 (ISBN 0 11 691611 7).

K Hinds and J R Gregory. *National Diet and Nutrition Survey: children aged 1½ to 4½ years. Volume 2: Report of the dental survey.* London: HMSO, 1995 (ISBN 0 11 691612 5).

B Holland, A A Welch, I D Unwin, D H Buss, A A Paul and D A T Southgate. *McCance and Widdowson's The Composition of Foods*. 5th ed. Cambridge: Royal Society of Chemistry and Ministry of Agriculture, Fisheries and Food, 1991 (ISBN 0 85186 391 4).

Supplements to the above:

A A Paul, D A T Southgate and J Russell. *Amino acids, mg per 100 g food, fatty acids g per 100 g food*. The first supplement to *McCance and Widdowson's The Composition of Foods*. London: HMSO, 1980 (ISBN 0 444 80220 7).

S P Tan, R W Wenlock and D H Buss. *Immigrant foods*. The second supplement to *McCance and Widdowson's The Composition of Foods* (4th ed.). London: HMSO, 1985 (ISBN 0 11 242717 0).

B Holland, I D Unwin and D H Buss. *Cereals and cereal products*. The third supplement to *McCance and Widdowson's The Composition of Foods* (4th ed.). Nottingham: The Royal Society of Chemistry, 1988 (ISBN 0 85186 743 X).

B Holland, I D Unwin and D H Buss. *Milk products and eggs*. The fourth supplement to *McCance and Widdowson's The Composition of Foods* (4th ed.). Cambridge: The Royal Society of Chemistry, 1989 (ISBN 0 85186 366 3).

B Holland, I D Unwin and D H Buss. *Vegetables, herbs and spices*. The fifth supplement to *McCance and Widdowson's The Composition of Foods* (4th ed.). Cambridge: The Royal Society of Chemistry, 1991 (ISBN 0 85186 376 0).

B Holland, I D Unwin and D H Buss. *Fruit and nuts*. The first supplement to *McCance and Widdowson's The Composition of Foods* (5th ed.). Cambridge: The Royal Society of Chemistry, 1992 (ISBN 0 85186 386 8).

B Holland, A A Welch and D H Buss. *Vegetable dishes*. The second supplement to *McCance and Widdowson's The Composition of Foods* (5th ed.). Cambridge: The Royal Society of Chemistry, 1992 (ISBN 0 85186 396 5).

B Holland, J Brown and D H Buss. *Fish and fish products*. The third supplement to *McCance and Widdowson's The Composition of Foods* (5th ed.). Cambridge: The Royal Society of Chemistry, 1993 (ISBN 085186 421 X).

W Chan, J Brown and D H Buss. *Miscellaneous foods*. The fourth supplement to *McCance and Widdowson's The Composition of Foods* (5th ed.). Cambridge: The Royal Society of Chemistry, 1994 (ISBN 0 85186 360 4).

W Chan, J Brown, S M Lee and D H Buss. Meat, poultry and game. The fifth supplement to *McCance and Widdowson's The Composition of Foods* (5th ed.), Cambridge: The Royal Society of Chemistry, 1995 (ISBN 0 85186 380 9)

W Chan, J Brown, S M Church and D H Buss. Meat products and dishes. The sixth supplement to *McCance and Widdowson's The Composition of Foods* (5th ed.), Cambridge: The Royal Society of Chemistry, 1996 (ISBN 0 85404 809 X).

A Mills and H Tyler. *Food and Nutrient Intake of British Infants Aged 6–12 months*. London: HMSO, 1992 (ISBN 0 11 242906 8).

Ministry of Agriculture, Fisheries and Food. *Fatty acids*. The seventh supplement to *McCance and Widdowson's The Composition of Foods* (5th ed.) Cambridge: The Royal Society of Chemistry, 1998 (ISBN 0 85404 819 7).

Ministry of Agriculture, Fisheries and Food. *National Food Survey*. Annual reports of the National Food Survey Committee. London: The Stationery Office (Reports previously entitled *Household food consumption and expenditure*).

Ministry of Agriculture, Fisheries & Food. *Food portion sizes*. London: TSO, 1993 (2nd ed.) (ISBN 0 11 242961 0).

Ministry of Agriculture, Fisheries and Food. *Dietary and nutritional survey of British adults; further analysis*. London: TSO, 1994 (ISBN 0 11 24296 1).

M Nelson, M Atkinson, J Meyer. Food Portion Sizes: A Photographic Atlas. MAFF, 1997.

J Steele, A Sheiham, W Marcenes, A Walls. *National Diet and Nutrition Survey: people aged 65 years and over. Volume 2: Report of the oral health survey.* London: The Stationery Office, 1998 (ISBN 0 11 243017 9).

Index

Printed in the UK for TSO
106234 02/05 C15 10170